Physicians and Social Change

Physicians and Social Change

JOHN COLOMBOTOS
Columbia University

CORINNE KIRCHNER
American Foundation for the Blind

New York   Oxford
OXFORD UNIVERSITY PRESS
1986

Oxford University Press

Oxford New York Toronto
Delhi Bombay Calcutta Madras Karachi
Petaling Jaya Singapore Hong Kong Tokyo
Nairobi Dar es Salaam Cape Town
Melbourne Auckland

and associated companies in
Beirut Berlin Ibadan Nicosia

Published by Oxford University Press
200 Madison Avenue, New York, New York 10016

Oxford is a registered trademark of Oxford University Press

Library of Congress Cataloging-in-Publication Data
Colombotos, John.
  Physicians and social change.
  Bibliography: p. Includes index.
  1. Social medicine—United States. 2. Physicians—United States—
Attitudes. I. Kirchner, Corinne. II. Title. [DNLM: 1. Attitude
of Health Personnel. 2. Delivery of Health Care—United States.
3. Role. 4. Social Change. W 62 C718p]
RA418.3.U6C65 1986   362.1'72'0973   85-18954
ISBN 0-19-503685-9

Printing (last digit): 9 8 7 6 5 4 3 2 1

Printed in the United States of America
on acid-free paper

To Katina, Yanna, Elias, and Peter
and
Betsy and Kathy

Foreword

The organization of medical care in the United States is undergoing a major transformation. Some factors influencing change have evolved over relatively long periods, such as the dynamic growth of bio-medical science and technology, the aging of the American population and escalating costs of medical care and publicly sponsored medical care programs. Others—such as the anticipated oversupply of physicians, the rapid growth of for-profit hospital chains, new ambulatory services and surgi-centers, and increased competition among innovative organized plans—are of more recent vintage, not until relatively recently on the forefront of health policy discussions. Many physicians face this new environment with a sense of opportunity, uncertainty, and anxiety.

The profession of medicine has been a dominant force in defining and controlling the nature of medical work. Emerging conditions make it inevitable that it increasingly will share its influence and autonomy with corporate and insurance plan managers, government regulators, and organized consumer groups. But it would be naive to assume that the enormous power of the profession, painstakingly and skillfully cultivated over this century, will be quickly or substantially reversed despite changing conditions and the growing pool of competing physicians. Physicians will continue to affect substantially the patterns of medical care, appropriate standards, and the costs associated with varying episodes of illness. They certainly will do so under greater constraints, but there proletarianization is hardly inevitable.

We have many images of the physician, typically shaped by the issues of the moment, the mass media, and our individualized experiences. These in turn reflect the public and visible stance taken by organized medicine and spokespersons for varying specialties, subspecialties, and other professional interest groups. These images typically convey a fairly monolithic view of doctors and fail to capture the heterogeneity of the half-million physicians in terms of social background, political and social orientations, work settings, and generational cohort. Nor do they convey the potential adaptability or resistance of varying groups of physicians to different types of public and private initiatives.

Over the past decade many surveys have been conducted of physicians' attitudes and opinions about issues on the public agenda. But these studies are overwhelmingly descriptive and typically lack either a conceptual perspective or sufficient depth to convey the complexity of influences that motivate doctors and shape their views of public issues or the nature of their work. In this book, John Colombotos and Corinne Kirchner present the results of a comprehensive survey and sophisticated assessment of physician reactions and their determinants. Building on long-standing conceptual perspectives in the social sciences, and carefully linking their work to the studies of others on physician behavior and related issues, they dissect clearly and informatively the wide array of personal, socio-political and work influences that shape doctors' orientations. Using a national sample of physicians, house officers, and medical students surveyed in 1973 and a longitudinal study of doctors in New York State covering the periods prior to and following the enactment of Medicare, they examine among many other issues how the anticipation of public programs, and their enactment and implementation, influence how doctors respond.

If this were simply a typical study of the attitudes of doctors it would be of passing historical influence. Because Colombotos and Kirchner focus on generic issues in contrast to description, their concepts and analysis have as much relevance to the emerging debates as to the issues of the time. Any cross-sectional study is limited, of course, in types of inferences possible. But the richness of the analysis, and the careful manner in which questions are framed, not only yields much that is important and provocative but also serves as a useful model for future studies of physicians and other occupational groups.

The authors inquire, for example, about effects due to generational differences among doctors as compared to those resulting from professional aging irrespective of birth cohort. Moreover, they inquire how important historical events such as the enactment of Medicare affect response irrespective of cohort or age. Throughout they are sensitive to the fact that social life involves a continuing process of selective sorting in which people seek contexts consistent with their needs, aspirations, and values. Thus, while examining the effects of socialization on the attitudes of medical students, residents, specialists, and fee-for-service versus salaried group practitioners, they also consider the effects of self-selection.

This book offers a variety of surprises that challenge common views of the profession of medicine. In 1973 majorities of physicians favored group practice over solo medicine and were agreeable to fixed fees. When National Health Insurance (NHI) seemed inevitable, as it did in 1973, most physicians had accommodated to the idea of at least some form of NHI. As the authors point out quite elegantly in their analysis of physician response to Medicare, doctors accept the inevitable, particularly if their basic interests are not violated. While in 1964 only a minority of doctors supported Medicare, shortly after it was passed, but before doctors had much experience with the program, almost three-quarters were in favor. As physicians actually experienced Medicare in action they became strong supporters and staunch defenders of its benefit structure. A key conclusion to be taken from the authors' analyses is that the level of support or opposition to major initiatives at a particular point may be less important than the force of a social and political consensus, and that physicians will accommodate if their vital interests are not violated.

This study finds many differences among physicians depending on background characteristics, comparable to differences often found in the general population as well. It also identifies variations by generation, by specialty, and by practice setting. In intriguing analyses, the authors suggest that physician attitudes are characterized by considerable "pluralistic ignorance," a lack of awareness that other doctors share their "progressive" views to the real extent they do. Also, they demonstrate that leaders of organized medicine are remarkably in tune with their membership despite frequent commentary to the contrary. At least in recent years the American Medical Association has struggled to keep within one organization physician groups varying substantially in their economic interests and political ideologies. Physicians have been more divided than ever before and their interests commonly clash. With a growing surplus, such competing interests are likely to be even more acrimonious. If experience as captured by Colombotos and Kirchner is prologue to the future, we can anticipate considerable efforts on the part of the AMA to moderate differences and to seek to define issues that unify their diverse physician constituencies.

Akin to other studies that penetrate beyond the surface of public affairs, this analysis also shows vividly the complexity of physician attitudes. Physicians' political views have an important influence on how they view government involvement and a variety of organizational and economic issues and thus they are not simply "professional" matters. But many of the issues that concern doctors are specific to the processes of developing their skills and standards, and providing effective care to patients; in these areas doctors are less likely to be divided by their politics.

There has been much speculation about the future of the medical profession and the erosion of traditional physician autonomy. At varying times the agent of threat was seen to be government, or academic physicians, or managers of large "medical empires." The present locus of fear among many is the large medical corporation with its focus on the bottom line and its concern with profitability for its shareholders. There seems little doubt that the mix of "regulation," "competition," and entrepreneurship we are presently experiencing will have fundamental influences on how care is organized, where it is given, and the mix of procedures and services. But it is also important to remember, as this study clearly shows, that the profession of medicine, contrary to stereotype, is extraordinarily heterogeneous and highly adaptive. There will be major realignments in influence and payment, but the resilience of doctors as individuals, and as organized groupings, will no more easily succumb to the power of the corporation than it did to the power of big government. The corporations have lesser constraints than government, but they too will have to maintain the trust of physicians and the public. The physician's image is somewhat more tarnished than in past years but should times get really tough there remains a store of public good will they can call upon, particularly if they are perceived as speaking in the public interest and not solely in their own.

Rutgers University   David Mechanic

Preface

When I began the research reported in this book in the nineteen sixties, a number of studies of the organization and policies of the American Medical Association were in print. In contrast, little was known about the attitudes and opinions of the nation's "rank-and-file" physicians toward political and health care issues.

This led me to conduct a study of New York State private practitioners in 1964. The passage of Medicare a year later provided a unique opportunity for a natural experiment on the effects of legislation on physicians' attitudes toward Medicare and related issues. Reinterviews with physicians in the 1964 sample were conducted at three points in time after the passage of Medicare, through 1970. By this time Corinne Kirchner had joined me on the project. In 1973 the New York State study was extended to include national samples of physicians in all types of activities and settings (in office- and hospital-based practice, medical teaching, administration, and research) as well as interns and residents and medical students. This expanded the analysis of subgroup differences in the attitudes of physicians and permitted an examination of the publicized "generation gap" in medicine in the early nineteen seventies.

The purpose of this book is to analyze how physicians differ among themselves and how they change in their attitudes toward broad political questions and basic issues in the organization of health care, such as practice arrangements, peer reviews, task delegation, methods of physician reimbursement and payment, and the role of government in health care. Despite a decline in the power of the medical profession in recent years, it continues to be a significant force in the politics of health care and what physicians think and what they do make a difference in how the health care system works.

The book offers an analysis grounded in a number of key sociological and social-psychological concepts rather than a purely descriptive report, thus minimizing the "datedness" of the data. Among these concepts are attitude structure, pluralistic ignorance socialization through the life cycle, age-generations, law as an instrument of social change, and oligarchy in voluntary organizations.

Physicians' attitudes toward specific issues are discussed in relation to their attitudes toward broader issues, issues that persist into the present. The concept of *attitude structure*, the idea that attitudes tend to be related to other attitudes and to be embedded in a set of values, is critical to the analysis. We examine, for example, the extent to which physicians' attitudes toward health care issues are politicized, that is, related to their political views.

Socialization refers to the processes by which people acquire the values and attitudes of groups they belong to. These processes are grounded in socially patterned experiences characteristic of different groups. Differences in physicians' group memberships and socialization experiences are viewed as major sources of variation and change in their attitudes.

In research on the professions, the concept of socialization has often been introduced to study the development of orientations in relation to clinically relevant topics, such as attitudes toward certain types of patients, uncertainty, and "detached concern." Also, the use of the concept has generally been limited to studying experiences in formal training settings and has stressed the uniformity of the effects of such experiences.

In this book, the idea of socialization is extended to neglected nonclinical topics, namely political issues and changes in the organization of health care, and to neglected sources of socialization. The latter include both early, pre-training experiences, as reflected in physicians' *social* characteristics, such as socioeconomic and religious-ethnic background and gender, and later, post-training experiences, as reflected in physicians' *professional* characteristics, such as their practice setting and specialty. Thus, physicians' social and professional characteristics are viewed as indicators of socialization experiences that make for variation in physicians' attitudes; and the question of whether personality or current social environment is more important in shaping people's attitudes and behavior is reformulated to ask whether *earlier* or *later* social environments and experiences (early nurture vs. later nurture) are more important.

Historical events are also viewed as socialization experiences in order to analyze change in physicians' attitudes. While physicians' social and professional characteristics point to experiences according to their location in the social structure, their age-generation and their exposure to historical events point to experiences according to their location in the historical process. We examine the effects of Medicare as a case study of the effects of legislation on attitudes and behavior.

Finally, we come back full circle to a question that implicitly generated this research: does organized medicine represent the medical profession? We compare leaders, members, and nonmembers of organized medicine with respect to their social and professional characteristics, their attitudes, and the extent to which they feel represented by the American Medical Association.

This book has been written for several audiences: for teachers, researchers, and students in the social sciences and in public health and for health care policy makers and administrators. We hope it adds to the understanding of why physicians think and act as they do in a changing health care system.

New York   J.C.
November 1985

Acknowledgments

The interviewing for the studies on which this book is based was done by the National Opinion Research Center (NORC) of the University of Chicago. I would like to thank Paul Sheatsley, who was then with the New York office of NORC, for encouraging me to experiment with the telephone interview method, then relatively untried, when other experts were advising me that hour-long telephone interviews with busy medical practitioners "would never work"; Margot Karp, Lucille Kolkin, Doris Newman, and Pearl Zinner of the NORC New York office for their help in developing and testing the interview schedule and for their meticulous execution of the field work; Mary Foster, Cathy Charles, and Michael Millman, who were doctoral students at the time, for their active and stimulating participation as research assistants on the project; Regina Loewenstein for consultation in designing the national sample; Chris Theodore, Gene Roback, Louis Goodman, and Lynn Jensen of the American Medical Association staff for selecting the 1973 samples of physicians, housestaff, and medical students, and for providing useful AMA research publications and policy materials; the California Medical Association for providing data, before their publication, on its survey of California medical graduates; Elmer Struening and Gerhard Raabe for advice on constructing attitude scales and on the use of factor analysis; Bruce Link for his invaluable advice on the data analysis and for his detailed review of the entire penultimate draft with a special eye to conceptual and methodological issues; Samuel Bloom, Jack Elinson, Eugene Feingold, Raymond Fink, William Frucht, Bradford Gray, and Robert Zussman for their critical comments on the draft or on papers and chapters that survived their way into this book; Michele Ochsner for expanding and revising the section in Chapter 2 on "Problems and Trends in Health Care" and the section in Chapter 8 on "Politics and

Health Care Since the Mid-Seventies: Continuity and Change" and for her suggestions for reorganizing Chapter 8; Tom Fenn for taking on the computer during the terminal phases of the study; Amy Taylor Pfeils for her secretarial and editorial help on an early draft of the book and for suggesting an early version of the title; Hannah Frisch for her incredibly sustained and near-flawless effort at the typewriter and at the word processor, while at the same time ministering to the many needs of others in the Division of Sociomedical Sciences, Columbia University School of Public Health; Phyllis Starner, who, as administrative coordinator in the Division, takes on tasks that go far beyond those connoted by her title, and thereby makes it possible for books like this to get written; and Jack Elinson, the first head of the Division, who introduced me to the idea that the social sciences have something useful to say about health and health care problems and who encouraged me to pursue my interest in doing research on the medical profession.

The research on which this book is based was supported by the National Center for Health Services Research (NCHSR), Grant Number HS 00117. I thank NCHSR staff members Jerry Weston, Sherman Williams, Jere Wysong, John Gallicchio, and especially Jean Carmody, for their criticisms of various drafts and papers and for their support.

I also thank the publishers of the American Sociological Review for their permission to reprint portions of the article "Physicians and Medicare: A Before-After Study of the Effects of Legislation on Attitudes" (volume 34, June, 1969, pp. 318–334), which appear in Chapter 6.

I thank Jeffrey House, editor of the Oxford University Press, for his guidance and good-humored support in seeing the book through to its completion; Wendy Keebler and Ellie Fuchs, also of the Oxford University Press, for their gentle, but firm and efficient, shepherding of the pre-edited manuscript through to publication; and David Lane, for preparing the index.

Finally, I am deeply grateful to Lois Grau for her criticisms and for her sustained (and, on occasion, unrelenting) support and encouragement.

Contents

Physicians and Social Change

1 Introduction

It is impossible to understand the problem of medical care without understanding the physician. And it is impossible to make significant changes in the medical field without changing physician behavior.
Victor R. Fuchs (1974)

In 1969 President Nixon publicly recognized a "massive crisis" in health care in the United States. The components of that "crisis" were strikingly similar to the problems of health care delivery reported by the Committee on the Costs of Medical Care nearly fifty years earlier: the cost of health care, its accessibility, and its quality (Committee on the Costs of Medical Care, 1932). Those problems are no less salient in the eighties than they were a decade and a half ago, though cost has overshadowed accessibility and quality as the dominant concern.[1]

Proposed solutions to these problems reflect ongoing changes in the health care system. They have involved the role of government in the financing and organization of health services; the organization of health care services, such as group and hospital-based practice; reviews and controls of physicians' performance; the division of labor in health care, such as the use of nurse-practitioners and physicians' assistants; how physicians are reimbursed—by salary, capitation, fixed fees, or customary fee-for-service; and how consumers pay for care, including prepayment, co-insurance, and deductibles. These issues represent accelerating trends affecting the everyday professional behavior of physicians. They have been, and continue to be, hotly debated inside and outside of the medical profession.

The positions of organized medicine on these changes are generally well known. Little, however, is known about the thinking of the nation's individual physicians. The objectives of this book are to examine how individual physicians' attitudes toward these political and health care issues vary among different generations and subgroups of the profession and how they change.

The general aim of the book is to add to the understanding of the role of the medical profession in the nation's health care system, both in terms of the attitudes and behavior of individual physicians and in terms of the role of organized medicine. Underlying this aim is our conviction that the medical profession continues to be a critical participant in the shaping of the health care system; that what physicians think and what they do make a difference in how that system works and in how it evolves. The research reported here is thereby linked to broad historical and sociological analyses of the power relations between the professions and society and the politics of professionals (see, e.g., Dibble, 1962; Lipset and Schwartz, 1966; Freidson, 1970; Johnson, 1970; McKinlay, 1973; Ehrenreich and Ehrenreich, 1977; Larson, 1977; Brint, 1985).

Our empirical analysis of physicians' attitudes is guided by two concepts. First, people's attitudes are not isolated from one another. They tend to be related. How and to what extent are empirical questions. We view health care issues as, in part, political issues. Whether physicians consciously see them that way is problematic. In any case, we anticipated that physicians' attitudes toward health care issues would be statistically related to their political views; that is, that their health care views would be "politicized."

Second, we view physicians' socialization experiences as a major source of variation and change in their attitudes toward political and health care issues. Thus, we conceive of the social and professional characteristics of physicians (e.g., their socioeconomic and ethnic origins, the setting in which they work, and their specialty) as indicators of social experiences that directly or indirectly influence their attitudes. We address the question: What are the relative effects of physicians' early social origins and their later and current professional characteristics on their attitudes? In short, which is more important—early nurture or later nurture?

We also view historical events as socialization experiences. Whereas the social and professional characteristics of physicians point to experiences according to their location in the social structure, their generation and their exposure to historical events (e.g., the passage of Medicare) point to experiences according to their location in the historical process.

Methods

The data come mainly from two studies—one a longitudinal, telephone interview study of New York State private practitioners between 1964 and 1970 to measure the effects of the passage of Medicare on physicians' attitudes (Chapter 6), and the other, a national study of physicians and medical students in 1973.

In the New York State study, 1,535 private practitioners were interviewed altogether, 828 of whom were interviewed three times—once just before Medicare was passed (Time 1), a second time just before Medicare was to go into effect (Time 2) *or* six months after it went into effect (Time 3), and again five years after Medicare was passed (Time 4). Included in the 1,535 respondents were a control sample of 330 physicians interviewed at Time 2 to test for interview effect: 278 of this control sample were reinterviewed at Time 4. (A more detailed description of the longitudinal sample is given in Chapter 6.) A subsample of 142 office-based practitioners in New York State in the 1973 national study provides a "Time 5" measure, although it is not a part of the longitudinal sample.

In the 1973 national study, an expansion of the earlier New York State study, responses to telephone interviews or mail questionnaires were obtained from nationally representative samples of physicians and medical students. These consisted of 2,713 "senior" physician respondents (i.e., those beyond housestaff training) in all categories of professional activity, 1,303 interns and residents ("housestaff"), and 3,414 medical students in a representative sample of 24 medical schools. (Also, special samples of senior physicians included 576 medical faculty from 11 of the 24 schools from which the medical students were selected and 307 physicians in two large prepaid group practice plans. A more detailed description of the national samples is given in the section on "Sampling Designs" in the Appendix.)

Experimental comparisons of telephone and personal interview methods in the New York State study and of telephone interview and mail questionnaire methods in a pretest of medical students and housestaff in the national study showed no appreciable differences in responses according to these methods (Colombotos, 1969a; see section on "Data Collection Procedures" in the Appendix).

In this book, the data in Chapters 2, 3, 4, and 7 are based on the 2,713 senior physicians in the 1973 national study; the data in Chapter 5, on generational differences, are based on medical students, housestaff, and senior physicians in the 1973 study; and the data in Chapter 6, on changes in physicians' attitudes toward Medicare, come from the longitudinal study of New York State private practitioners.

The plan of the book is as follows:

In Chapter 2 we discuss those problems that make up the nation's health care crisis—the cost, quality, and accessibility of health care—and major long-term changes in the organization of health care. Our purpose here is to explain briefly how important trends—the participation of government in health care; group and hospital-based practice; reviews of practitioners' performance; a complex division of labor involving the delegation of "physician" tasks to nonphysicians; the reimbursement of physicians by salary; and prepayment—are related and how they may be viewed both as antecedents and as solutions to the health care crisis.

Our explication of these issues and a brief review of the positions taken by organized medicine introduce our description of physicians' attitudes toward the issues and their political views. These are the dependent variables in our research. The attitudes of physicians are compared with those of the public, where data on the latter are available. Finally, we analyze how physicians' political and health care attitudes are related and explain the crucial role of the idea of structure in the analysis that follows.

In Chapter 2 we describe our main dependent variables: physicians' attitudes. In Chapter 3 we describe a set of independent variables: physicians' social background characteristics (socioeconomic, ethnic, religious, regional, and national origins, and gender) and their professional characteristics—main activity (patient care, teaching, research, or administration); organization of work of those in patient care (individual practice, group practice, or hospital-based practice); method of reimbursement (salary, capitation, or fee-for-service); and specialty. We then compare the social backgrounds of physicians with those of the general population as evidence of selection into the profession; we describe trends in physicians' social backgrounds and professional characteristics as evidence of changes in the social composition and structure of the profession; and we describe how the background and professional characteristics of physicians are related.

In Chapter 4 we examine the socialization framework that links the social and professional characteristics of physicians to their attitudes. But we also consider alternative mechanisms, such as social selection and self-interest, which may explain the relationship between statuses and attitudes. We then examine the relative importance of physicians' early, social characteristics and later, professional characteristics on their attitudes toward different types of issues.

Whereas in Chapters 2, 3, and 4 we examine the *diversity* of physicians' attitudes in relation to their social and professional characteristics, in Chapters 5 and 6 we focus on *change* in these attitudes. The widely publicized "generation gap" in American medicine and the differences between more broadly defined generations are examined in Chapter 5. We view a generation, following Mannheim (1952: 291), as a group sharing a "certain characteristic mode of thought" because of location in "the social and historical process."

In Chapter 6 we examine the short-term effects of a major, more circumscribed historical event—the passage of Medicare—on the attitudes of the entire medical profession. The question is embedded in a more general issue: What is the role of law as an instrument of social change? We continue, in Chapter 6, to examine the conditions under which individual physicians changed their attitudes toward Medicare, including their prior attitudes toward other political and health care issues before the law was passed, and the extent to which changes in attitudes toward Medicare "generalized" to attitudes toward other political and health care issues. In comparing the reactions of physicians to Medicare and Medicaid in New York State, we conclude Chapter 6 with a discussion of the conditions under which different legislated health care programs are likely to influence physicians' attitudes and behavior.

In Chapter 7 we turn to a question implicit in our discussion so far: Does organized medicine represent the medical profession? Here we compare leaders at the AMA level and leaders, members, and nonmembers at the level of state and county medical societies regarding their social background and professional characteristics; their attitudes toward political and health care issues; and whether they feel represented by the AMA. Michels's classic analysis of organizational characteristics that lead to oligarchy is background to this analysis.

In the final chapter we summarize our main findings, review changes in politics and health care in the past decade, and discuss the implications of findings from our research and from more recent studies for current and emerging health care policies and programs.

Notes

1. Another concern expressed in the seventies was the growing "impersonality," "dehumanization," and "depersonalization" of health care, traceable to medical technology, specialization, and the bureaucratization of health care (Mechanic, 1972; Howard and Strauss, 1975). One hears little about this problem in the eighties.

2 The Ideology of the Medical Profession

In order to understand the core issues that form the substantive content of physicians' attitudes examined in this book—political ideology and government participation in health care, group practice, peer reviews, the delegation of tasks to nonphysicians, salaried reimbursement for physicians, and prepayment—we begin this chapter by reviewing the problems that make up the nation's health care crisis. Next, we discuss the major interrelated trends in the organization of health care over the past half century. Some of these trends may be viewed as antecedents of the health care crisis; others, as consequences. In both cases, we view these trends as issues, in the sense that they are controversial.

In conclusion, we discuss briefly the policies of organized medicine toward these issues; the attitudes of physicians and how they compare with those of the public; and, finally, how the attitudes of physicians are related to each other.

Problems and Trends in Health Care

The Health Care Crisis

The main components of the health care crisis, as we noted in Chapter 1, are the cost of health care, its accessibility, and its quality.

Cost

By the mid-1970s, uncontrolled and accelerating health care expenditures were already a central focus of concern (Fuchs, 1974; Knowles, 1977). Even a cursory examination of trends in health care costs reveals why.[1] In

1950, $10 billion were spent on personal health care (physician services, hospital stays, nursing home care, drugs, and related services); in 1965, over $40 billion; and in 1975, $130 billion. Over those years the proportion of GNP allocated to health care grew from 4.4 to 8.6 percent. Health care costs continue to rise: the 1982 allocation for health care was $322.4 billion, or 10.5 percent of the GNP. When Medicare was passed in 1965, federal officials projected that its cost might reach $8.8 billion by 1990, 25 years later. In fact, that amount was surpassed within *seven* years; by 1983 Medicare costs stood at $60 billion (Wohl, 1984; USDHHS, 1982: 153). Price inflation, which in recent decades has consistently outpaced the annual growth of general consumer prices, has been an important factor in escalating costs. Other key factors include the growth and aging of the population as well as changes in the intensity and nature of health care services and in the organization and financing of medical care (Weichert, 1981; U.S. Congressional Budget Office, 1979; Somers, 1982).

Physicians are not accustomed to weighing costs as a factor in treatment. Until recently, they have been taught to strive for extraordinarily high degrees of diagnostic certitude without regard for the costs of high-powered technology and staffing patterns (Reilly and Legge, 1982). Because it is estimated that physicians directly influence 80 percent of all health care expenditures, the role of the physician is a necessary focal point for cost-containment strategies (Fuchs, 1974; Roemer, 1982).

Access

The problem of limited access to medical care takes many forms: sheer unavailability of services in some geographic areas, including sparsely populated rural areas as well as populous but poor inner-city areas; an imbalance between specialty and primary care; economic and cultural barriers; long waits before an appointment can be made to see a physician; and long hours in the waiting room.

Large geographic disparities exist in physician-to-population ratios: in 1976, South Dakota had 81 practicing physicians per 100,000 population compared to New York's 185 per 100,000 (Hanft, 1981). Physicians and dentists, particularly specialists, are most available in affluent states and metropolitan areas (Milio, 1975: 68–70). Overspecialization is also a barrier to comprehensive and coordinated health care services (Fuchs, 1974: 68–69; Hanft, 1981: 80). By 1975, over 60 percent of physicians were practicing in a nonprimary care specialty (Hanft, 1981).

Geographic and program barriers are frequently intertwined with financial, social, and psychological impediments to obtaining medical care. Despite their greater needs for care, the poor and the elderly are most likely to be constrained by these factors and have been labeled the "out-casts" of the medical care system (Milio, 1975). Public health insurance programs have to a large degree brought these outcasts into the main-stream of the medical care system: Medicare and Medicaid are credited with equalizing physician visits and hospital stays for the poor and nonpoor. By 1975, the poor visited physicians 18 percent more frequently than the nonpoor; lower income children visited physicians as frequently as those from higher income families (Davis and Schoen, 1978: 41–42). But when levels of disability are taken into account, there are indications that the poor still receive less care for their illnesses than the affluent (Dutton, 1978). Persons of low income are less likely to have a regular source of care or to receive preventive services such as prenatal care, childhood immunizations, and screening for breast or cervical cancer (Davis, Gold, and Makuc, 1981).

More general problems of access, not restricted to particular popula-tion groups, apply to certain types of services, including primary care, emergency care, and home care (Fuchs, 1974).

Quality

A number of problems are embedded in the concept of the quality of health care. "High quality" health care for all citizens has often been voiced as a national goal, but defining, measuring, and achieving quality have proven elusive. Rough approximations for measures of quality, such as measures of "structure" (e.g., number of hospital beds or physi-cians per 1,000 population) or "process" (e.g., prenatal care received, operations performed) have been substituted for more direct measures of the "outcome" of medical services on the population's health.

Many observers have begun to question the value of allocating addi-tional dollars to health care (Fuchs, 1974; Benham and Benham, 1975; Wildavsky, 1977). Studies in the mid-1970s revealed that while utilization of health care services had increased following the enactment of Medicare and Medicaid, the effect of these programs on the population's health status was far from evident (Chase, 1977; Elinson, 1977; Lerner and Stutz, 1977; Mooney, 1977; and Wilson and White, 1977). In defense of the longstanding public health goals of improved access, equity, and quality of care, other analysts emphasize the caring rather than curing function of medical services and note that the most frequently used indicators of the population's health status are insensitive measures of the values of medical care (Elinson and Siegmann, 1977; Starr, 1978; McDermott, 1980).

While the contribution of medical care to the population's health has become an increasingly controversial issue over the past decade, there are coexisting concerns about quality as judged in terms of adequate professional standards and the efficacy of specific technologies and procedures. Well-publicized charges of incompetent medical practice and unnecessary surgery have made quality an issue even for routine, medical practice, and too little is known about the effects of specific procedures. According to a report by Congress's Office of Technology Assessment, the efficacy of 80 to 90 percent of the medical procedures in use has never been scientifically established (U.S. Congress, Office of Technology Assessment, 1978). Attention has focused increasingly on the need to evaluate medical technologies for safety and efficacy. Marketing new drugs and medical devices requires FDA approval, but new medical and surgical procedures are not subject to routine evaluation before they are widely adopted. Many experts view a more systematic program of technology assessment as important not only to meet quality concerns but also to aid in cost-containment (Altman and Blendon, 1979; U.S. Congress, Office of Technology Assessment, 1982).

These, then, are the interrelated components of the "health care crisis." Since the mid-1970s cost has become more central. A 1984 *New York Times* editorial declared: "Cost containment is the dominant issue in American health care" (May 14, 1984, p. A14). All components—cost, access, and quality—are affected, however, by changes in the organization of health care that have been ongoing since at least the turn of the century.

Trends in Health Care

The changes in the nature and organization of health care that we discuss briefly are:

1. the increasing specialization of health manpower and changes in the division of labor and expansion in the number and types of nonphysician personnel
2. the increasingly formal organization of medical practice, with group and hospital-based practice replacing individual practice
3. the financing of medical care through third-party payment
4. the reimbursement of physicians, with salary and fixed fees replacing customary fee-for-service
5. regulation and controls, including reviews of physicians' performance
6. the expanding role of government

Each of these trends generates a set of issues. It is physicians' attitudes toward aspects of these issues that are the focus of this book.

Specialization of Health Manpower

Fueled by the expansion in knowledge and technology—and in turn adding to its growth—health care has become increasingly differentiated.[2] Specialization has exploded within such established occupations as medicine and nursing, and it appears in the broader division of labor in health care in the form of a proliferation of new occupational groups. It also appears among such health institutions as hospitals that limit their services to specific levels of care (primary, secondary, tertiary, or aftercare) or to specified groups in the population (children, women, aging); and in the form of specialized services within institutions (e.g., neonatal intensive care units, burn centers, and trauma centers).

Within medicine, the trend toward specialization has been startling (Kendall, 1971: 449–525; Stevens, 1971). In 1923, barely 10 percent of the nation's physicians identified themselves as full-time specialists; by 1964, the figure had climbed to nearly 70 percent; and by 1981, to more than 90 percent (Somers and Somers, 1961: 29–30; Health Information Foundation, 1964; American Medical Association, 1983a: 15).[3]

The process is potentially limitless with the development of new specialties and the burgeoning of subspecialties in the interstices or within established, primary specialties, for example, neonatal-perinatal medicine, pediatric endocrinology, and gynecologic oncology.[4]

The proliferation of specialization within medicine has been paralleled by the proliferation of new occupations in health care. Whereas the ratio of physicians to all other health workers was 1:2 in the early 1900s, it is now approximately 1:15 (Ginzberg, 1983a). In 1978 there were 100 "allied health occupations and specialties," totalling nearly 1 million persons. These include laboratory workers and technicians, inhalation therapists, physical therapists, dietary workers, medical records personnel, and many others. In addition, there are nurses, who also have become increasingly specialized, and newer practitioner groups such as physicians' assistants and emergency medical technicians.

A major issue in this area is the appropriateness of substituting some of these personnel, most notably nurse-practitioners and physicians' assistants, for physicians in performing certain tasks (Barhydt-Wezenaar, 1981: 110–119). Arguments for physicians' delegation of tasks include potential cost-containment by using less expensive personnel; increasing physician productivity by relieving him or her of the more routine tasks; and access to more services than are available from physicians who do not delegate. Counterarguments include the possibility of higher cost, less personal relationships between physicians and patients, and less adequate care.

Group Practice

Although the traditional model of medical practice in the United States is the individual (solo) practitioner working out of his or her own office, roots of group practice go back to the turn of the century, when the famous Mayo Clinic was established.

Groups vary widely in a number of important characteristics: size, from three or four to over a thousand physicians; number and kind of specialties offered; proportion of participating physicians' income derived from fee-for-service or prepayment; mode of payment (straight salary, salary plus a share of net income, or "equal distribution"); and form of organization. (For recent data on these and other characteristics of group practice, see Held and Reinhardt, 1980; Phillips and Dorsey, 1980; American Medical Association, 1982a.)

The number and proportion of physicians in "bureaucratic" settings—group and hospital-based practice, health centers, and the like—have grown rapidly in recent decades. Although still a minority, the proportion of physicians in group practice has grown from only 1 percent in 1940, to 3 percent in 1946, 5 percent in 1959, 16 percent in 1969, and by 1980, to 26 percent (Somers and Somers, 1961: 40–41; Health Information Foundation, 1964: 2–3; American Medical Association, 1982a).[5]

Included in these developments has been the growth of prepaid group practice plans; for example, the Group Health Association, organized as a cooperative by and for government workers in Washington, D.C. in 1937; the Kaiser-Permanente groups, inaugurated by Henry Kaiser to provide health care for his factory workers in the early 1940s; and the Health Insurance Plan of New York, established in 1947.

How Physicians Are Reimbursed

Parallel to the bureaucratization of medical practice is the increasing proportion of physicians deriving all or part of their income from salaried arrangements. This trend is attributable in part not only to the growing number of physicians engaged mainly in nonpatient care activities (teaching, administration, research) but also to the increasing number of physicians who are in full-time group or hospital-based salaried practice or who have arrangements with hospitals and other institutions that provide a partial salary.

The proportion of physicians in "private practice" (defined as those who reported their principal employer as "self-employed") declined from 86 percent in 1931, to 75 percent in 1949, to 63 percent in 1964 (Health

Information Foundation, 1964: 1). In our 1973 national study sample, 30 percent of the senior physicians reported that they received all of their income in salary; and another 18 percent reported more than half of their income in salary.[6]

Financing of Medical Care

As out-of-pocket payment for hospitalization and even for many routine medical procedures has become less and less affordable for most families, third party mechanisms for spreading the cost of care have become increasingly important. Between 1929 and 1975, the proportion of medical expenses covered by some form of health insurance rose from 12 to 67 percent (USDHHS, 1982: 139). Although estimates differ, between 80 and 92 percent of the population is currently covered to some extent by some form of health insurance (Margolis, 1981; USDHHS, 1985). Although private health insurance underwrites roughly one-quarter of all health care expenditures, government programs, most significantly Medicaid and Medicare, are responsible for 40 percent of all health care costs and constitute the largest single source of payment. Government not only directly insures the aged, disabled, and poor, but also indirectly subsidizes the purchase of private health insurance through tax deductions and tax exclusions for employer contributions to health insurance (U.S. Congressional Budget Office, 1982).

Nevertheless, significant gaps remain in the types of services covered by private and public insurance programs (Margolis, 1981). Mental health care, dental services, vision care, home care, preventive services, and drugs are among the types of health care expenses most frequently borne by consumers. The Medicare program covers only about 44 percent of total health care costs of the elderly (Iglehart, 1982b). Due to stringent eligibility requirements, only one-third of the "poor" qualify for Medicaid (Davis, Gold, and Makuc, 1981). Despite such limitations, third-party payments have become the financial underpinning of the health care sector, and, as the single largest payer, government has come to occupy an increasingly important role in defining the organization and nature of health care services.

Reviews and Controls

All components of the health care system—hospitals, nursing homes, insurance carriers, the pharmaceutical industry, and the medical profession—have been increasingly subjected to reviews and controls in recent decades. (Some prefer the term "regulation" in place of "reviews" and "controls.")

These trends have been spurred by the rise of third-party payers and by the increasing participation of government in the financing of health care. The goals of these interventions are containment of costs as well as improvement of quality and access. They include a wide variety of programs and practices, such as certificate-of-need laws, rate regulation, regulations for marketing a new drug, licensing (and relicensing) of health practitioners. Some are forms of "self-regulation," such as the accreditation of hospitals and professional schools and "peer reviews."

Physicians-in-training and physicians who taught or practiced in academic teaching hospitals in the past were no strangers to peer reviews, in the form of hospital rounds. In the late 1940s the American College of Surgeons extended the concept by establishing hospital tissue committees to see if operations were justified. In the early 1950s, the Joint Commission on Accreditation of Hospitals introduced medical audits to assess the quality of care in hospitals in terms of such measures as the rate of postoperative complications. And by 1974, after the enactment of the Professional Standards Review Organizations legislation, the Joint Commission had mandated medical audit programs as a basis for accreditation (USDHEW, 1976).

The first sustained utilization-review program, based on a retrospective analysis of hospital records by medical staff committees, was initiated in western Pennsylvania in 1959 by a group including Blue Cross, the county medical society, and the hospitals. This type of program spread rapidly to other parts of the country (Berman and Gertman, 1981: 44). Such a plan was later required for participation in Medicare and Medicaid. The Professional Standards Review Organizations (PSROs) program, enacted in 1972, is generally regarded as one of the major pieces of federal health legislation in the 1970s. It required that care provided to Medicare and Medicaid inpatients be reviewed by nonprofit associations of physicians to ensure that it conformed to "appropriate professional standards" and was "medically necessary." The program fizzled, however, because of lack of financial support by the federal government (Mihalski, 1984: 50). In the early eighties, PSROs were replaced by PROs (Professional Review Organizations), revived to keep tabs on the prospective reimbursement program (diagnosis-related groups, or DRG's) in hospitals (Mihalski, 1984: 51–53). "Second-opinion" programs, in which the need for elective surgery is re-examined by a board-certified specialist (without charge to the subscriber), were initiated by Blue Cross in the early seventies and have become common practice.

A recent countertrend—"deregulation"—notwithstanding, the general, long-term trends are clear. Various types of peer review programs, initiated by the government, other third-party payers, and accreditation bodies are no longer a rarity in medical practice. The trend is augmented by the increase in the number of physicians practicing in groups, hospitals, and other institutional settings, which provide the potential for, though they do not ensure the practice of, informal assessments of each others' performance. Many of these groups have voluntarily developed formal peer review programs. (For a description of such a formal program in a prepaid group practice plan, see Deuschle et al., 1982.)

The Role of Government in Health Care

The health care system in the United States is one of the few in which the balance of private versus public involvement is still weighted in favor of the former. Indeed, ours is the only "developed" country without universal government-sponsored health insurance. Lipset (1970) and Wilensky (1975), among others, have stressed the dominance of a conservative, laissez-faire political ideology as inconsistent with the growth of strong government action in the social welfare fields.

Traditionally, government responsibility in health care has been limited to care of the indigent. (For a review of the role of government in health care in the U.S., see Jonas and Banta, 1981.) In recent decades, however, government participation in a wide range of activities related to health—construction of facilities, biomedical research, education of health professionals, and financing of health care—steadily increased.

During this period the emphasis of federal health policy has gone through a series of transformations. In the 1950s, the major form of governmental involvement in the health care sector was through the Hill-Burton hospital planning and construction program. Through federal and state subsidies, Hill-Burton was a major stimulus for health facility expansion.

Also, during the post-World War II years, government involvement in basic medical research expanded dramatically, a shift with important consequences for medical education and practice. Prior to the 1930s, federally sponsored research was done in government laboratories, but with the passage of legislation establishing the National Cancer Institute (NCI) under the National Institutes of Health (NIH), new precedents were established: the Public Health Service was permitted to make grants to outside researchers and a program of training fellowships was created.

As other categorical institutes joined NCI, and, with strong lobbying efforts, medical research became a popular cause. The NIH budget grew at an astronomical rate: between 1941 and 1960, federal expenditures for medical research increased from $3 million to $400 million. By 1982, roughly $5 billion were allocated for this purpose (USDHHS, 1983).

With a new and redistributive agenda for domestic policy in the 1960s, governmental responsibilities in the health care sector became increasingly ambitious. Along with Medicaid and Medicare, a number of more limited health programs also appeared or expanded during the Johnson years, including Neighborhood Health Centers, Maternal and Child Health programs, and Community Mental Health Centers. Among these programs, only Medicare was administered directly. Government still exercised few direct controls (Lee and Estes, 1983; Marmor and Dunham, 1983).

National health insurance was considered inevitable in the early seventies, but was shelved around the middle of the decade. As the investment of governmental payers in health care increased, it was inevitable that government would increasingly attempt to shape the delivery of health care. By the early 1970s, it was generally recognized that Medicaid and Medicare had fueled the rapid escalation of health costs through open-ended cost-based reimbursement for hospital care and open-ended fee-for-service payment for physician services (Milio, 1975). The vast amount of money being poured into health care also failed to ensure full and equal access to services, high quality care, or appropriate distribution of facilities and personnel. To address these concerns as well as the issue of cost, new reviews and controls were enacted in the 1970s, notably, the PSRO legislation of 1972 that we mentioned earlier. Such reviews conflicted with unlimited physician discretion in decisions such as length of hospital stay or the use of costly technology and were widely viewed as the most significant legislation affecting the medical profession for decades.

A second major federal initiative, the Health Planning and Resources Development Act of 1974 (P.L. 93-641) was intended to address many pressing issues in health care including coordination of care, access, quality, cost, and unmet needs for preventive and mental health care services. The act required health facilities to obtain "Certificate of Need" approval from state health agencies before undertaking major capital expansion. It also created more than 200 local planning agencies charged with developing implementation plans that would be in line with federal goals (Marmor and Dunham, 1983).

Other important governmental initiatives include the Health Maintenance Organization Act of 1973 and a number of federal and state programs intended to control the growth of hospital costs. As the decade of the 1970s drew to a close, however, regulatory approaches to achieving health policy goals came increasingly under fire.

How Trends Are Related

These trends are connected in complex ways with each other and with each of the three components of the health care crisis described earlier. We will outline some of these relationships by identifying a few manageable clusters, starting with the effects of medical technology. (For similar attempts to trace the dynamics of these trends, see USDHEW, 1976: 405–409; Twaddle, 1982: 327–331.)

Medical Technology

The more there is to be learned and mastered, the greater the pressure to limit the breadth and to increase the depth of expertise, that is, to specialize. (The social-psychological pressures inducing medical students and practicing physicians to choose a specialty have been analyzed by Kendall and Selvin [1957], and Kendall [1971: 449–497].) On the institutional level, the effects of the accumulation of knowledge, of other cognitive intellectual factors, and of political and organizational forces (e.g., the size and concentration of social units) in spurring specialization in medicine has also been the focus of study (Rosen, 1944; Bucher and Strauss, 1961; Stevens, 1971; Kendall, 1971).

Conversely, specialization tends to expand the knowledge base, thus stimulating the creation of new technology. Technology sometimes operates to increase, and sometimes to reduce, the cost of health care. More, and costlier, things are done to extend the lives of many patients who otherwise would die. Patients may continue to depend on continuing high-cost technology for survival (renal dialysis is an example). On the other hand, advances in technology may result in cost-savings; for example, the long-term institutionalization of tuberculosis patients has been replaced by treatment with relatively inexpensive drugs. And other recent pharmacological advances have eliminated the need for more costly surgery. The net impact of medical technology, however, has probably been to increase the cost of health care.

Technology also affects the quality of care, again in a double-edged manner. It may prolong lives and enhance health status; but it also may have negative effects if used inappropriately, and it may raise profound ethical and legal questions about the quality of life.

Finally, technology spurs coordination and organization, both to create still newer technology and to facilitate cost-sharing arrangements for the more economical use of expensive equipment.

Specialization

Specialization affects the quality of care positively by more effectively applying medical knowledge to patients' problems. But it increases the cost of medical care by expanding the armamentarium of medical knowledge and skills and by duplicating services.

Specialization also demands social mechanisms for coordinating diverse activities, hence the need for organization. Mechanisms such as a referral system coordinate the activities of geographically dispersed practitioners (Freidson, 1979). Group practice and other forms of institutionally based practice go one step further by concentrating practitioners under one roof and by implementing more formal coordinating mechanisms such as administrative practices and a central records system.

Organization

Supporters of group practice attribute a number of advantages to this form of practice. They argue that it saves money by sharing the cost of facilities and equipment and by optimizing the use of ancillary personnel; and that it produces better quality care by making readily available a range of specialized skills, and, because the work of practitioners is relatively observable, by producing the potential—if not the actuality—of peer review and criticism.

When combined with prepayment and salaried reimbursement, prepaid group practice has, it is argued, additional advantages in reducing costs and improving the quality of care. By removing the economic barrier and thereby making preventive and early diagnostic care more accessible, prepayment substitutes less costly ambulatory care for costlier hospital care. By eliminating financial incentives inherent in fee-for-service, salaried reimbursement also cuts costs and improves the quality of care (Freidson, 1979). But group practice, it is conceded, may have disadvantages: some patients complain that it makes care more impersonal (Freidson, 1961).

Financing

Provided there are budgetary controls and cost-cutting incentives, as in a prepaid group practice plan, health insurance may cut costs. Alternatively, it may raise costs if there are no such controls and incentives. For example, Medicare has been singled out as a major cause of the rise in health care spending since the late 1960s.

But health insurance programs, financed by both governmental and nongovernmental sources, have shown an increasing concern with controlling costs, and they have exercised leverage to that end. The PSRO program and the second-opinion programs for surgery are examples.

The capability of health insurance programs to collect data and to monitor services (with the help of computerized records) has expanded their potential for reviewing both the cost of medical services and their medical appropriateness.

Government

The infusion of government funds in financing health care and biomedical research has set in motion a complex set of trends. In health care, it first drove up the cost of health care and then created pressures to control those costs and to assure quality through regulatory programs such as HSAs, PSROs, and HMOs. In biomedical research, it expanded medical technology, supported the expansion of academic medical centers, and added to the pressures for specialization.

It is plausible to expect that the interrelationships among these objective trends are reflected in the thinking of physicians about these issues— that is, in the structure of physicians' attitudes. We will see that this is the case in the latter part of this chapter.

The Policies of the American Medical Association

As we noted in Chapter 1, much has been written about the health care policies of organized medicine, particularly the American Medical Association, but relatively little about the attitudes of individual physicians, which are the substance of this book. The policies of organized medicine, however, are a significant part of the context in which the attitudes of individual physicians are embedded. (The extent to which organizational policies are congruent with "rank-and-file" physicians' attitudes, and how they may influence one another, are examined in Chapter 7.) We turn next to a brief overview of these policies.

We begin with two caveats. First, to most people "organized medicine" means the American Medical Association. But, just as the "medical profession" is differentiated in terms of individual physicians' social and professional characteristics (Chapter 3), which are in turn linked to their attitudes (Chapter 4), so, too, "organized medicine" is differentiated along lines corresponding to social and professional characteristics of physicians. Medical societies and organizations are based on geography (state, county, medical societies), gender, race, specialty, and patient care versus academic medicine. The policies of these groupings may differ, or even clash (see Chapters 7 and 8).

Second, the policies of these organizations, no less than the attitudes of individual physicians, change. In the early part of this century, the American Medical Association was known as a "progressive" organization. At that time it supported compulsory national health insurance (Numbers, 1978). By the early twenties, however, it had turned against NHI, and for the next half century the AMA assumed a general stance of opposition to most proposals for change in the organization of medical practice. By the early seventies, observers were noting another turn; they cited evidence of "bureaucratic adaptation" in the traditionally "recalcitrant" policies of the AMA (Tatalovich, 1971).

With these caveats in mind, we limit our summary review to the policies of the American Medical Association for three reasons: the AMA is the most inclusive organization of physicians; it is still the most powerful politically; and consequently, because its policies have been the most fully documented, it provides an adequate basis for analysis.

The policies of the American Medical Association over the past half-century can be most concisely represented as a defense of individual, fee-for-service practice free of any third-party involvement, especially governmental. Proposals for incremental change in the financing, organization, and delivery of health care—government participation in medical care, group practice, voluntary health insurance and prepayment by patients, salaried or capitation reimbursement for physicians, peer reviews, and task delegation—have all been consistently met by the AMA's initial opposition. That opposition is grounded in a code of ethics that defends the sanctity of the doctor-patient relationship, the quality of medical care, and the public good—and in appeals to "the American way." Impassioned critics, however, some within the medical profession, have labeled the AMA and its policies as reactionary, negative, and self-serving (Means, 1953: 140–183). More dispassionate investigators, such as economist Paul Feldstein, have examined the policies of the AMA in relation to its unstated goal of "maximizing the income of its members" (Feldstein, 1977: 27–75).

Consider these examples of AMA policies:[7]

In the early thirties, the *Journal of the American Medical Association* (*JAMA*), responded to the Committee on the Costs of Medical Care's support of group practice by referring to medical groups as "medical soviets." In *JAMA*'s words, "The alignment is clear—on the one side, the forces representing the great foundations, public health officialdom, social theory—even socialism and communism—inciting to revolution; on the other side, the organized medical profession of this country, urging an orderly evolution" (Editorial, *JAMA*, Dec. 3, 1932, p. 1950). The AMA also condemned voluntary health insurance. It changed its policy later in the decade when serious proposals for government-sponsored compulsory health insurance materialized ("The American Medical Association: power, purpose, and politics . . . ", 1954: 971–982).

In the late forties, compulsory national health insurance was labelled "socialized medicine," supported by "the President. All who seriously believe in a Socialistic State. Every leftwing organization in America . . . The Communist Party." "Compulsory Health Insurance is one of the final, irrevocable steps toward a regimented state . . . [It] isn't just a threat to health; it is a threat to freedom" (American Medical Association, *The Voluntary Way is the American Way* . . . n.d.).

In the fifties, *JAMA* condemned some types of salaried practice (the "corporate practice of medicine") as "unethical," arguing that under such an arrangement the primary loyalty of physicians would be to their employers rather than to their patients. The AMA feared that salaried hospital practice would lead to exploitation of the physician and a lowering of the dignity of the profession ("The American Medical Association: power, purpose, and politics . . . ," 1954: 978–979).

According to the AMA, criticism among physicians is to be avoided at all costs. A physician "should not disparage by comment or insinuation the one who preceded him [in treating a patient] . . . [such insinuation] tends to lower the confidence of the patient in the medical profession and so reacts against the patient, the profession, and the critic" (American Medical Association, 1969: 7). Government-directed peer review programs were especially objectionable. In 1980, the AMA House of Delegates voted to "encourage the elimination" of all such programs, including PSRO (American Medical Association, 1982b). Earlier, in the 1974 meeting, it had conceded that repeal of PSRO may have been "impossible to achieve," but had urged vigilance with respect to "the potential dangers in the areas of confidentiality, malpractice, development of norms, quality of care, and the authority of the Secretary of HEW" (quoted in Feldstein, 1977: 34). Blue Cross–Blue Shield "second-opinion" programs were also initially opposed by the AMA (Feldstein, 1977: 35).

The use of other health practitioners, such as nurse-practitioners and physician-assistants, in recent years has been monitored closely by the AMA. The issue is whether they should *substitute* for or *complement* the activities of the physician. The AMA has opposed independent practice by these personnel. Rather, physician control is assured by mandating, in the case of physician-assistants, that their services be "under the supervision and direction of a licensed physician who is responsible for the performance of that assistant." Reimbursement for these services would go to the employing physician (Feldstein, 1977: 46–49).

Most of these policies have been modified, some substantially. Group and salaried practice are now acceptable, if not preferred. The AMA proposed its own version of national health insurance (Medicredit) in the early seventies.

This is not to say that the AMA has turned around to spearhead a radical transformation of the American health care system. Rather, it has adopted a general policy of "symbolic adaptation" to a rapidly changing health care environment (Tatalovich, 1971: 114–130). Others have put it more bluntly: "new ideas which the Association has accepted have been forced upon it" ("The American Medical Association: power, purpose, and politics . . . ", 1954: 1022).

Some of these adaptations took place when continuing opposition appeared futile. The AMA has chosen to participate in programs it initially opposed in order to exercise *some* control and influence over their development rather than to remain outside—without a voice. For example, rather than a Medicare boycott, supported by a number of resolutions introduced at the AMA's House of Delegates in June 1965 as the bill was going through its final stages in Congress, cooler heads urged that the profession "actively participate" in the development of Medicare's rules and regulations and its actual implementation, working to "contain" and "amend" the legislation along the lines of the AMA's "Eldercare" program (Tatalovich, 1971: 116).

The AMA response to the PSRO program was remarkably similar. At the 1974 convention, the AMA House of Delegates stopped short of calling for repeal of the program. But it recommended that the AMA "direct its efforts to achieve constructive amendments to the PSRO law and to ensure appropriate regulations and directives . . ." (quoted in Feldstein, 1977: 34). In 1980, when the political winds had shifted, the AMA adopted a policy "to encourage the elimination of all government directed peer review programs, including PSRO" (American Medical Association, 1982b: 22).

In 1983, the AMA reaffirmed its opposition "to Peer Review Organization (PRO) programs by fiscal intermediaries or other third parties," but recommended "that state medical societies not already involved in the PRO program now consider involvement *to maintain physician direction*" (*emphasis added*) (American Medical Association, 1984: 40).

Other shifts in policy were apparently made to stave off more objectionable actions. As we noted earlier, it was only in the face of serious proposals for "governmental compulsory health insurance" in the late forties that the AMA espoused voluntary health insurance after doing "almost everything possible to prevent its development . . . through the 1930s and early 1940s" ("American Medical Association: power, purpose, and politics . . . ," 1954: 981–982). In the same spirit, the AMA proposed its own conservative version of NHI (Medicredit) in the early seventies when it seemed that one of a number of more progressive versions would be adopted.

In sum, despite changes in AMA positions, especially in recent years, in spirit it has continued a conservative policy on the political and health care issues discussed in this chapter. Against that background, we turn next to examine the attitudes of individual physicians.

Physicians' Attitudes Toward Political and Health Care Issues

Political Ideology and Government in Health Care

Interest in the political ideology of the professions and its implications for social change has a long history. The professions posed a difficult problem of classification in the Marxist conception of stratification, in which social classes were defined by their relationship to the means of production. Early writers on stratification and ideology speculated whether the professions were a liberal or a conservative force (see Ben-David, 1963–64: 247–50; Ehrenreich and Ehrenreich, 1977).

Generally, the professions are viewed as politically conservative. (The terms "liberal" and "conservative" in this discussion refer to "economic-welfare" issues involving the acceptance of government activity in solving social problems, such as poverty, unemployment, education, and health. "Non-economic" issues, such as race relations, civil liberties, international relations, and sexual mores, to which the terms "liberal" and "conservative" are frequently applied, are not included in this analysis.) The conservative ideology of professionals is consistent with Durkheim's view of professional organizations as preconditions of societal consensus and stability in a highly differentiated society (Durkheim, 1957). It is also consistent with the view that the political stance of professionals, like that of other groups in society, is dictated by self-interest, which means, in the case of privileged professionals, protecting the *status quo* (see Freidson, 1970; McKinlay, 1973). But, in fact, compared to business executives, professionals are more liberal on welfare state issues (see Brint, 1985).

A useful framework by Lipset and Schwartz (1966) suggests two general sources of variation in the political ideology of different professions: social stratification variables and distinctive values inherent in different professions. Since they are disproportionately drawn from upper socio-economic backgrounds and since they enjoy high social status and economic rewards, physicians might be expected to be more conservative in their thinking than other professional groups, and certainly more conservative than the general population.

On the other hand, the "humanistic ethos" of physicians may predispose them to their "relatively greater liberalism . . . among the more rewarded professions" (Lipset and Schwartz, 1966: 308). Also, the scientific orientation of physicians is presumed to temper their investment in preserving the *status quo*. "As members of a profession strongly committed to science, physicians must learn professional values which are inconsistent with political conservatism" (Glaser, 1960: 241).[8]

Yet the medical profession is commonly believed to be among the more conservative groups in society. (A possible source of this belief is discussed in Chapter 7.) Indeed, for Parsons, it is a paradox why a profession which is "organized about the institutionalization of applied science" and thus expected in general "to be in the forefront of the general process of 'progressive' change in industrial society should politically align itself with the elements which have been resisting these very patterns of change" (Parsons, 1963: 33).

Although the medical profession is often portrayed as monolithically conservative in its political views, we found that a considerable number of physicians do not fit this mold. Asked how they identify themselves in their "political thinking" (Q.90), a majority called themselves either "liberal" (23%) or "middle-of-the-road" (37%); another 37 percent called themselves "conservative."[9] (Only 1% saw themselves on the "radical left" and another 1% on the "radical right.") Moreover, although the majority (58%) considered themselves "Republicans" or leaning toward the Republican party, nearly a third (31%) considered themselves "Democrats" (Q.88A) or leaning toward the Democratic party.

With respect to general "economic-welfare" issues, physicians are generally conservative. Only about a quarter gave liberal responses, that is, "agreed" with each of four items that made up an "economic-welfare liberalism" scale (see Appendix for a description of this and other scales), such as: "It is the responsibility of society, through its government, to guarantee full employment" (Q.34H); "The government should play a bigger part in the economic life of the nation in order to distribute income more equally" (Q.34I); "Poverty could almost be done away with if we made certain basic changes in our social and economic system" (Q.34J); and "The United States needs a complete restructuring of its basic institutions" (Q.34K). (Physicians' responses to all of these questions on "political" issues discussed in this section were highly intercorrelated, as we shall show later in this chapter. Self-identified liberals tended to be Democrats, to take liberal positions on economic-welfare issues, to favor NHI, and so on.)

The distributions of physicians' responses take on more meaning, however, when they are compared with similar data from the general population or from other professional or occupational or socioeconomic groups, especially those whose income and education are similar to those of physicians. We discuss such comparisons in a later section of this chapter.

Government in Health and Medical Care

We expected physicians' acceptance of the involvement of the federal government in various areas of health (Q.20) to vary according to the activity in question. Most acceptable, we anticipated, would be federal involvement in constructing hospitals, in medical school curricula, and in biomedical research, while federal involvement in providing medical care to poor people, in physicians' specialty choices and practice locations, and in regulating the drug industry would be relatively unacceptable. Our expectations were based on our reading of AMA policies on each of these issues.

The findings were surprising. "Providing medical care to poor people" was by far the most acceptable (81% thought the federal government should be involved in it "a great deal" or a "fair amount"); less acceptable—though still with majority approval—was "regulating the prescription drug industry" (61%), influencing "where doctors practice, by giving scholarships" (54%), and constructing hospitals (52%). Less acceptable were setting "priorities in biomedical research" (45%) and shaping "students' choice of specialty, by giving scholarships" (35%); least acceptable was influencing "medical school curricula" (only 15%). We considered the possibility that the relative acceptability of the activities varied with the extent of actual federal involvement, but such a pattern does not seem to hold.[10]

Turning to general issues in medical care, physicians ranged widely in terms of whether they gave "conservative" or "liberal" responses. Whereas 70% of the physicians agreed that "regardless of shortcomings, the United States health care system is the best in the world," a "conservative" view, nearly an equal number (64%) agreed that "it is the responsibility of society, through its government, to provide everyone with the best available medical care, whether he can afford it or not," and nearly half (44%) did not think that "decisions about the organization of health care should be entirely in the hands of the medical profession," both of which are "liberal" views.

Physicians' attitudes toward various dimensions of Medicare and national health insurance, which are indicators of their attitudes toward the more general domain of the role of government in medical care, were examined in some detail.

MEDICARE. A large majority (82%) of the nation's physicians were "in favor" of Medicare (Q.12) in 1973, eight years after its passage. And, although half (47%) thought that Medicare "goes just far enough," more than a third (37%) believed that "Medicare does not go far enough in providing medical care for older people"; only 9 percent thought that "it goes too far" (Q.14).

Furthermore, physicians were divided in their perceptions about other consequences of Medicare. Nearly two out of five (38%) thought that "most doctors [were] earning more money under Medicare," and only 5 percent, "less money"; just over half thought that Medicare had made no difference or had no idea about its effects on doctors' income (Q.17). Half (49%), however, thought that Medicare had affected "the individual doctor's professional freedom" either "a great deal" or "a fair amount" (Q.18). Physicians' perceptions and attitudes toward Medicare, passed in 1965 and implemented in 1966, changed radically over a six-year period beginning just before its passage, as we shall see in Chapter 6. In any case, physicians' perceptions and attitudes toward Medicare in 1973 contrasted sharply with their perceptions and attitudes toward NHI.

NATIONAL HEALTH INSURANCE. The NHI debate had evolved during the early 1970s beyond the point of merely discussing *whether* a program should be enacted to *what type* of program. As noted earlier, the AMA brought out its own proposal, "Medicredit," to answer more liberal NHI bills. The AMA's reaction was reminiscent of its response to the imminence of Medicare, when it unveiled "Eldercare," in early 1965. "Eldercare," like "Medicredit," relied on the principle of government subsidies for the purchase of private health insurance policies.

Attitudes toward the General Idea of NHI and Perceptions of Colleagues' Attitudes: A case of pluralistic ignorance. Three-fourths (74%) of the physicians interviewed thought that most of the doctors they knew personally were opposed to "some form of national health insurance"; only a fifth (19%) thought that most were in favor (Q.32). Yet, when asked about their own attitudes, more than half (56%) were in favor of some form of NHI (Q.22).[11]

We found the same pattern of discrepancy between physicians' own attitudes and their perceptions of their colleagues' attitudes toward Medicare, though that discrepancy narrowed over time. In May 1966, after Medicare was passed, 70 percent of private practitioners in the State of New York were in favor of Medicare, but only 26 percent thought most of their colleagues were in favor of it. In January 1967, six months after Medicare's implementation, 81 percent were in favor, while 58 percent thought that most other doctors were in favor, and in April 1970, when 92 percent were themselves in favor, 81 percent thought that most other doctors were in favor of Medicare. The attitudes and perceptions of New York State practitioners stabilized at this level through 1973 (in the national study), when 91 percent favored Medicare and 78 percent thought that most other doctors were in favor.[12]

These perceptions and attitudes are strongly correlated: 91 percent of those who perceived that most of their colleagues were in favor of NHI were themselves in favor of it, compared with less than half (46 percent) of those who perceived that their colleagues were opposed to it. Do perceptions influence attitudes, or do attitudes influence perceptions? Probably both processes occur. People's perceptions of the attitudes of others may influence their own attitudes toward an issue. This is the essence of mutual influence. On the other hand, physicians may attribute their own attitudes to their colleagues. Also, physicians who favor NHI, for example, are probably more likely than physicians who do not favor NHI to number among their acquaintances physicians who *in fact* favor NHI.

However, how does one explain the pronounced *underestimate* by physicians of support for NHI among their colleagues? The discrepancy between the *actual distribution* of attitudes toward NHI and perceptions of this distribution is a classic instance of "pluralistic ignorance," a situation in which an individual member of a group *assumes* that he/she is virtually alone in holding certain attitudes and expectations, not knowing that others privately share them (Merton, 1957: 377; Breed and Ktsanes, 1961: 382; O'Gorman, 1975). According to Merton, this condition is frequently observed in a group so organized that *mutual observability* among its members is slight. (It may be that pluralistic ignorance varies among different subgroups of physicians according to such structural characteristics of their work settings as observability and the degree to which they are integrated into formal and informal colleague networks.)

It has been noted that pluralistic ignorance has a conservative bias. In their analysis of the public's attitudes toward desegregation in a southern city, Breed and Ktsanes postulated that the error of people in estimating the actual distribution of opinion tended "to favor the older existing beliefs in the system rather than the direction of change" (1961: 383). Here is a clue to explain the discrepancy between the attitudes of physicians toward Medicare and NHI and their perceptions of their colleagues' attitudes. It is possible that physicians ascribe views to their colleagues that are in line with what they perceive to be the historically conservative policies of the AMA. In other words, they assume that the AMA "speaks for" other doctors, if not for themselves. We return to this issue in Chapter 7, where we speculate about why the AMA is perceived to be more conservative than it may be in fact.

Inevitability of NHI. More than four-fifths of the physicians believed—in 1973—that some form of NHI was *inevitable*; nearly three-fifths expected it within five years (Q.23A). Physicians were not alone in anticipating the coming of NHI. As we mentioned earlier, the public debate about NHI had evolved by then beyond the point of *whether* a program should be enacted to *what type* of program.

How are the *beliefs* of physicians about the inevitability and imminence of NHI related to their *attitudes* toward NHI? Among those who saw some form of NHI as inevitable within one year, fully 88 percent were in favor of it, compared with 70 percent of those who saw NHI as inevitable within the next two or three years, and so on, down to only 23 percent in favor among those who believed that NHI was *not* inevitable. We conceive of the belief in the inevitability of NHI, as an "anticipatory fait accompli" (see Chapters 6 and 8).

Expectations of Effects of NHI. Although physicians had limited knowledge about NHI (nearly half reported that they were either "not well informed" or "not at all informed" about the various proposals), at the same time they ventured to indicate their expectations about the effects of a hypothetical compromise NHI plan on their own work and on the health care system. Their expectations were generally negative. A majority (55%) expected at least a "fair amount" of unnecessary hospitalization (Q.31D); even more (76%) expected at least a "fair amount" of unnecessary use of doctors' services (Q.31E). Two-fifths (42%) predicted there would be a decline in the quality of medical care (Q.31C). Three-fourths (77%) expected at least a "fair amount" of federal interference with the professional freedom of doctors (Q.31G) compared with, as noted earlier, a half (49%) who thought that Medicare had affected the professional freedom of individual doctors that much. A quarter (27%)

thought that "most doctors would . . . earn less money," and only 14 percent, "more money" under NHI (Q.31F), compared with only 5 percent who thought that "most doctors [were] earning . . . less money" under Medicare, and 38 percent who thought "more money."

As we shall see in Chapter 6, private practitioners in the State of New York were much more negative in their expectations of the consequences of Medicare *before* its implementation than they were in their perceptions of its consequences *after* implementation. Comparisons, therefore, between physicians' judgments of the consequences of Medicare and of NHI—in 1973—should take into account that the former had been in effect for seven years while the latter—NHI—had not been legislated.

Here again, returning to NHI, those physicians with negative expectations were generally less likely than those with positive expectations to favor the general idea of NHI, with one exception: physicians' expectations of the effects of NHI on the incomes of doctors were unrelated to their attitudes toward the general idea of NHI.

This contrasts with Medicare. Physicians who thought that most doctors were earning *more* money under Medicare were much more likely to favor Medicare than those who, in turn, thought it made no difference and those who thought most doctors were earning less money. This contrast between Medicare and NHI is tantalizing. A clue is offered when we note the absence of a relationship between income expectations and perceptions and attitudes toward Medicare among private practitioners in the State of New York in 1966, just before implementation, and subsequently in 1967 and in 1970. (We do not have data on physicians' expectations before the passage of Medicare.) It is possible that physicians' perceptions of the impact of a program on their incomes become linked to their attitudes only after they know more about it or have had considerable experience with it.

Group Practice

The theoretical and practical problems posed by "independent" professionals working in bureaucratic organizations has received considerable attention. Although some norms are shared by the professional and bureaucratic models of work—impersonality, a division of labor based on technical expertise, and emphasis on the application of knowledge—one view stresses inherent conflicts between the two. The norms of independent professionals are seen as clashing with bureaucratic rules and hierarchy (Ben-David, 1958: 255–274; Blau and Scott, 1961; Scott, 1966).

An alternative view stresses the mutual adaptation of the two models

(Litwak, 1961; Scott, 1966; Barr and Steinberg, 1980); hierarchical supervision gives way to collegial relations dictated by rules of etiquette (Freidson, 1975), or at most, to a system of informal advice (Goss, 1961).

The dominant ideology of medical practice in the U.S. is the antithesis of that of bureaucratic organization. It stresses a rugged individualism in medical decision-making (see Freidson's discussion of the "clinical mentality," 1970: 158–184; and Colombotos, Kirchner, and Millman, 1975a) as well as in the organization and management of physicians' day-to-day practice. That the ideological model bears little resemblance to the de facto organization of even individual practice has been aptly described by Freidson (1979: 297–307).

The central problem, identified by Hughes (1955), is:

> Given current trends in medical organization, it [is] . . . important to discover not merely the extent to which the go-it-alone [individual practice] model prevails as against the team-work [group practice] model, but also to find out *what influences continue to reinforce it. (Emphasis added)*

Features of group practice compared with those of individual practice that are commonly believed to attract physicians include more regular hours, paid leave and vacation time, a stable income, the professional stimulation of colleagues and opportunities to keep abreast of the latest in medicine, access to consultation and advanced medical technology, and the opportunity to practice high-quality medicine. Features that deter physicians include a ceiling on income, possibly poor relationships with colleagues and patients, and the restriction of individual initiative (see MacColl, 1966; Donabedian, 1969; Fink, 1980; Wolinsky, 1982).

Although, as we shall see in Chapter 3, considerably less than half (37%) of the study sample were in an individual or partnership practice, more than half (57%) believed that a small group practice of three to five physicians was "likely to lead to the best medical care" (Q.35A). A large group practice was the second most likely, in physicians' judgment, to lead to the best medical care (chosen by 25%), far outdistancing individual practice (7%) and a partnership of two physicians (4%). Physicians' preferences among these arrangements as "most desirable" for themselves, assuming that their income were the same, were roughly parallel to their choices based on quality, except that slightly more named an individual and partnership practice as "preferred" than named them as "best."

Individual practice was indicated as the "least desirable" form of practice (Q.35C) by 43 percent of the physicians—more than those who identified a large group based in a hospital (31%) and a large group not based in a hospital (16%). A partnership, a single-specialty small group, and a multispecialty small group were each indicated as the least desirable by only 2 percent.

Thus, a sizable number of physicians in this country practice in arrangements other than those that they believe lead to the best medical care and that they would prefer when they were asked to *assume income were not a factor.* It would appear that income was a factor in their responses, or that there were constraints on their ability to choose their preferred settings.[13]

Peer Reviews

The medical profession, like all professions, resists lay control over the technical work of its members. It asserts that it polices itself through peer review and that external controls are unnecessary. This is the essence of the claim to professional autonomy. It is the recognition of this claim by society that distinguishes the professions from other occupations (Freidson, 1970).

In recent years, however, there has been growing public debate about whether the professions, including medicine, are in fact willing or able to regulate their members. The escalating use of public funds for health services in this country has led to legislative concern about "accountability," although it is not always clear what is meant by "accountability" and how it should work (Rivlin, 1971: 121; Etzioni, 1975: 121–142).

In an influential paper on the professions, Goode argued that peer review—without public disclosure—is "functional" both for individual professionals and for the larger society, which benefits from the professionals' expertise (1957: 198–199):

> In exchange for protection against the larger society, the professional accepts the social control of the professional community.
>
> As a consequence the larger society has obtained an *indirect* social control by yielding *direct* social control to the professional community, which thus can make judgments according to its own norms . . .
>
> Professional life is so fundamentally based on achievement, that such judgments of rank are made constantly . . .
>
> [However] structural factors in the interaction between the professional community and the larger society suggest that the evaluations, which are the daily experience of all professionals, cannot and will not be formalized and made public.

Goode's theoretical propositions are implicitly based on two empirical generalizations: (1) that peer reviews are a part of the daily experience of professionals, and (2) that, furthermore, "the professional accepts the social control of the professional community."

A contrasting view is Freidson's analysis of the profession of medicine (1970: 137–184; 1975). Freidson argues that physicians generally resist reviewing, and being reviewed by, their colleagues. Even in a model setting providing high potential for effective peer reviews—namely, a multispecialty, prepaid group practice in a university-affiliated hospital, staffed by "exceptionally well-trained, experienced physicians," all board-certified or board-eligible—he found that the operating norms (the "rules of etiquette") "limited the critical evaluation of colleagues' work and discouraged the expression of criticism" (1975: 241).

Goss (1961) observed a similar reluctance by physicians to engage in formal peer judgment in a setting that seems even more conducive to peer reviews, the outpatient clinic of a large teaching hospital. When physicians did comment on each other's work—even when the reviewer was in a superior faculty or hospital rank—it was given as informal "advice" rather than as an "order," and was indicated on a slip of paper *clipped to* the chart rather than as an official entry *in* the chart.

These strategic studies by Freidson and Goss suggest that even where the structure of practice permits review, physicians are reluctant to criticize the work of their colleagues and to take action. (For a systematic inquiry into the laxness of the profession in exposing and prosecuting misconduct, see Derbyshire, 1969.) Greater reluctance is expected among solo practitioners: on the average, they are less credentialed, they may feel less self-confident professionally, and the relatively low visibility of solo practice may attract physicians who are especially sensitive to criticism; in turn, solo practice may nurture this sensitivity.

Physicians' resistance to review and criticism, argues Freidson, is grounded in their "clinical mentality," which he defines as composed of several factors: an emphasis on personal responsibility to individual patients rather than to an aggregate (i.e., a community) and on firsthand clinical experience rather than on scientific laws or general rules; a crude pragmatism that emphasizes results rather than abstract theory; a tendency to take action for its own sake and to believe in the efficacy of what one is doing; and a sense of uncertainty, risk, and vulnerability to being wrong (1970: 158–184).

These tendencies are viewed as stemming from the "nature of medical work." They are reinforced by emphasis on individual autonomy and independence, stemming from physicians' predominantly middle- and upper-class origins.[14]

Conscience Versus Reviews

There are two broad philosophical alternatives about how to ensure high-quality professional performance: one is a "collectivist" orientation that emphasizes reviews and controls by professional peers or by public regulation; the other is an "individualistic" orientation that emphasizes reliance on practitioners' "conscience" (individual self-regulation).

Moore vividly discusses the potential conflict between the two views (1970: 130).

> An *occupation's* claim to self-regulation, which is a kind of collective assertion of autonomy, has a doubtful relation to the *individual* autonomy of the professional . . . If the autonomy of the group is made the basis of a kind of private police state—which happens in some local medical societies—then we have to reconsider the meaning of autonomy. Organization and licensing may be made the basis of a *genteel terror* . . . Collective autonomy and individual autonomy may turn out to be inconsistent goals. Identification with peers may become subservience to peers, and that ends the effective sense of *personal responsibility.* (*Emphasis added*)

In response to a survey question about these broad alternatives, most physicians (77%) in the national study expressed an individualistic orientation by agreeing with the statement: "A doctor's conscience is more important for the quality of medicine he practices than are reviews of his work by other doctors" (Q.34F).

This finding indicates widespread agreement with the AMA's premise that the key determinant of high performance is the "character," or "conscience," of the physician. Basic character formation occurs well before medical school, and, therefore, the crucial concern is *selection* of the right types of persons to enter medicine: "Every physician should aid in safeguarding the profession against admission to it of those who are deficient in moral character or education" (American Medical Association, 1969: 19).

Attitudes Toward Different Types of Reviews

Physicians' resistance to reviews varies according to what *types* of reviews are being considered.

A typology of reviews would include the following dimensions:

1. *What aspects* of performance are being reviewed—for example, what skills, what kinds of patients, in what settings?
2. *How* are the reviews conducted, that is, what *mechanisms* are used?
3. *By whom* are the reviews conducted?
4. *For whom* are reviews conducted and *what action* is taken?

Here we examine physicians' responses to only a few questions about reviews, specifying *settings* (hospital vs. office practice) and *auspices* (under national health insurance).

REVIEWS IN DIFFERENT SETTINGS: HOSPITAL VERSUS OFFICE. Peer review procedures were initially institutionalized primarily in hospitals. Tissue committees have been increasingly augmented by other types of ongoing medical audits required by the Joint Commission on Accreditation of Hospitals and by government-financed programs, as under PSRO's and PRO's.

Asked about peer reviews in hospitals, the great majority (83%) of the physicians responded favorably (Q.39). In sharp contrast, when asked about "reviews of doctors' work in their *offices* by other doctors," the proportion in favor dropped to less than half (48%) (Q.40).

REVIEWS UNDER NHI. Seventy-five percent of the physicians preferred a national health insurance plan "under which the work of doctors is routinely reviewed by a panel of practicing doctors" rather than a plan without such a system of reviews (Q.26). This surprisingly high level of support for peer reviews under NHI could be due to ambiguity in the question: the alternative could be taken either to mean an NHI plan with *no* formal reviews whatsoever or a plan with reviews by physicians who were *not* in practice, or even by nonphysicians. We assume that one reason the proportion of physicians who preferred the peer review option was so high is that some respondents preferred reviews by practicing physicians rather than by physicians *not* in practice, if there were to be reviews at all.

Delegation of Tasks

A cornerstone of the medical profession's control over the terms and organization of its work lies in its control over the medical division of labor (see Rayack, 1967: 240–272; Freidson, 1970: 47–70; Feldstein, 1977: 50–57), which gives it the power to limit, direct, and determine the work of other health occupations.

The general reluctance of physicians to delegate to other health workers tasks commonly associated with doctors' work is easy to understand in light of its claim in staking out an area of *exclusive* technical competence. A realignment of tasks could strike at the heart of this claim.

The resistance of physicians to task delegation, however, is likely to vary according to certain attributes of those tasks. Specifically, we expect greater resistance to the delegation of tasks that require, or are perceived to require, a great deal of judgment; that have a high probability of a mistake or serious consequences from a mistake; that are new and relatively untried; and that cannot be direclty supervised (see Levy, 1966: 50–54).

We found that nearly two-thirds (64%) of the physicians in the national study responded that they would hire a nurse-practitioner or a physicians' assistant, assuming they were "properly trained" and working under the physician's supervision (Q.38).

As expected, however, there was wide variation in the duties that physicians were willing to delegate to such persons (Q.37). Whereas 91 percent agreed that it is appropriate to delegate "counselling a diabetic patient about his diet," only 8 percent thought it was appropriate to delegate "differentiating between functional and organic murmurs."

In general, physicians were least willing to delegate tasks that involve *judgment*, such as in *diagnosis* ("diagnosing throat conditions" [32% would delegate], "reading simple chest x-rays in a screening program" [32%], and "differentiating between functional and organic murmurs" [8%]), and in *decisions about what data to collect* ("deciding what allergy tests to do" (23%]).

They were *most* willing to delegate tasks that involve:

- the *routine collection of data* ("taking preliminary histories" [84%], "doing allergy tests" [78%], "doing routine well-baby followups" [72%], and "doing routine prenatal checkups on the mother" [65%]); and
- *routine treatment* ("counselling a diabetic patient about his diet" [91%], "doing minor suturing" [76%], and "performing uncomplicated deliveries in the hospital" [53%]).

There was considerable variation in the acceptability of delegating tasks within each of these broad categories, however, and considerable overlap between them. Performing "routine physical examinations," unspecified and on cardiac patients, would be delegated by only 39 and 22 percent, respectively, and "treating superficial corneal abrasions" would be delegated by only 26 percent, even though they involve "routine" procedures or a "superficial" condition.

The delegation of "decision-making" tasks apparently depended on the specific problem presented. Several decisions—"if suturing is necessary" (would be delegated by 61%), whether a patient with a "minor complaint" should be seen by a doctor (by 62%), and prescribing medication for minor pain relief (by 60%)—were relatively acceptable; while one—whether to prescribe an antibiotic for a sore throat (19%)—was relatively unacceptable.

Methods of Physician Reimbursement

Several years ago, I made it a practice to ask every physician whom I met in connection with my work the following question: "What do you think of the suggestion that all physicians should receive a regular salary?" The replies were always the same, namely, "What amount of salary did you have in mind?" (C. Rufus Rorem, 1954, cited in Somers and Somers, 1961: 51)

As we noted earlier, increasing numbers of physicians work under a salaried arrangement. The image of the salaried doctor, however, is still regarded by some as a specter to be avoided. Skeptics and cynics may say that the only objection of doctors to salary is economic self-interest, based on the assumption that a straight salary is likely to yield lower income than is possible from fee-for-service practice, as suggested by Rorem. However, both supporters and opponents of the idea of paying doctors by salary have predicted *non*economic consequences. On the one hand, it is argued that a salary means loss of professional independence and also weakens the doctor's personal ties to his patients and the incentive to practice high-quality medicine. On the other hand, it is argued that an assured salary frees doctors from considering economic gain in their relations with patients, thus avoiding unnecessary procedures and sky-rocketing costs. A salaried arrangement, the argument continues, permits physicians to concentrate on purely medical matters. Clearly, the issue of method of physician remuneration has both ideological and economic self-interest components.

The attitudes of physicians toward various methods of reimbursement were obtained from questions linked to national health insurance. Physicians were asked (after a series of questions about various aspects of NHI): "a question about how doctors should be paid under national health insurance. Would you be agreeable or not agreeable to . . . a plan under which all doctors are paid an *annual salary*?"

Similarly, they were asked whether or not they would be agreeable to a plan under which "family doctors would be paid an annual amount per patient" and a plan under which "all doctors" would be paid a "fixed fee for each service" and "their own customary fees for each service" (see Q.28).

Not surprisingly, *customary fee-for-service* was most acceptable, agreeable to three-quarters of the physicians. A surprisingly high level of support for fixed fees was expressed, however; 61 percent of the doctors said they would be "agreeable" to an NHI plan under which all doctors would be paid a "fixed fee for each service, negotiated by a committee on which physicians are represented." A quarter (24%) of the physicians felt they could agree to an annual amount for each patient, while only 14 percent agreed to an annual salary.

Note that physicians were not asked which method they *preferred*. Preference and acceptability converge when we consider how many doctors said only *one* method would be "agreeable." Except for customary fees, the numbers who were agreeable to only one of the other methods were negligible. Among the combinations, the following were the main groups:

- those who would be agreeable *only* to customary fees (28%), the most conservative position with respect to physician reimbursement
- those who would be agreeable to customary fees *and* to fixed fees, or to fixed fees only, but not to capitation or salary (40%)
- those who would be agreeable to various other combinations involving customary or fixed fees *and* capitation or salary (26%)[15]

Returning to the issue of economic self-interest, the majority (64%) of the physicians in patient care (to whom the question was restricted) believed that they would earn the highest income under customary fees, followed by fixed fees (13%), capitation (6%), and an annual salary (4%) (Q.29). The ordering corresponds to the acceptability of the reimbursement options.

Prepayment

As we noted earlier in this chapter, the proportion of medical care financed by some form of insurance (or "prepayment") has risen steadily since the 1930s to a point where more than 80 percent of the population is currently covered in varying degree by some form of health insurance. Initially, the AMA fought the movement for voluntary insurance covering hospital care in the 1930s on the grounds that it would eventually lead to inclusion of physicians' services and to "compulsory insurance under government control." It was right on both counts. Organized medicine has adapted, however, to the growth of insurance covering both hospital and physician services. And physicians are quite receptive to prepayment mechanisms.

Asked which of a series of payment mechanisms they preferred "assuming that the physician gets paid a fee for each service," only 4 percent chose prepayment that provides "complete care to a family for a flat sum in advance" (Q.36); but a small minority, 16 percent, chose traditional fee-for-service in which the patient is not reimbursed. A third (36%), however, chose a "modified prepayment" plan in which the patient pays a "small fee—say a dollar or two—for each service," and an equal proportion (38%) chose an indemnity plan in which "the patient pays for each service and is completely reimbursed by a third party."[16]

Physician Versus Public Opinion

We alluded earlier to the more conservative general political views of physicians compared with those of the general population. In response to questions worded similarly, but not identically, to ours, 30 percent of the general population (in 1974) called themselves some shade of "liberal" ("extremely," "slightly," or just "liberal"), compared to 23 percent of our physician sample; and 30 percent called themselves some shade of "conservative," compared to 37 percent of our physician sample. With respect to political party preference, the difference was larger: 56 percent of the general population identified with the Democratic party, compared to 31 percent of physicians, while 33 percent of the general population identified with the Republican party, compared to 58 percent of physicians (National Opinion Research Center, 1980).

These differences generally persist with respect to their views about the role of government in health care and other aspects of health care delivery:[17]

The public and physicians differed sharply with respect to Medicare before its passage. Between 60 and 65 percent of the American public favored Medicare during the period 1961–65 (Schiltz, 1970: 171), compared to less than 20 percent of the medical profession (*Medical Tribune*, May 15, 1961).

The public and physicians differed less with respect to NHI—in 1978: 64 percent of the public felt there "was a need for national health insurance," compared with 53 percent of the medical profession. By 1981, however, the gap had widened because support for NHI remained stable among the public (68% still supported it) whereas it dropped to 30 percent among physicians (American Medical Association, 1981a: 16; 1981b: 70).

The HMO concept and "the use of nurse practitioners, midwives, and physicians' assistants" were more likely to be "very" or "somewhat acceptable" to the public (to 61% and 63%, respectively) than to physicians (to 40% and 43%, respectively) in 1983–84 (Louis Harris and Associates, 1984: 34, 36).

The public and physicians differed in their overall assessment of the health care system (in 1983–84): only a fifth (21%) of the public thought "the health care system works pretty well, and only minor changes are necessary to make it work better," compared to nearly half (48%) of physicians (Louis Harris and Associates, 1984: 7).

And, finally, physicians were much less likely than the public (in 1983–

84) to accept such options as government price controls on doctors' and hospital fees and diagnosis-related, group-based fixed fees (DRG's) (Louis Harris and Associates, 1984: 31–36).

In sum, physicians are more conservative than the general public on a wide range of political and health care issues, the size of the gap depending on the specific issues raised and on the historical period. Physicians may be no more conservative than those in other high-income occupations, however. Controlling for income, they were more likely than lawyers, for example, to be Democrats (cited in Lipset and Schwartz, 1966: 308). And a 1972 Carnegie Commission study of faculty in American universities showed that those in medicine were close to the middle in their political views. They were more conservative than those in social work, the social sciences, the humanities, law, and the fine arts, but more liberal than those in agriculture, business, and engineering (Ladd and Lipset, 1975: 62–64, 77–79). Whether these differences between occupations occur among nonacademics as well as among academics is, of course, open to question.

The Structure of Physicians' Attitudes

Physicians' attitudes and beliefs toward various components and aspects of each of the sets of issues that we have discussed tend to be correlated, as we noted earlier in this chapter. Thus:

- Various measures of political attitudes—self-identifications as liberal or middle-of-the-road or conservative; political party preferences; and attitudes toward economic-welfare issues—are strongly related.
- Physicians' attitudes toward different components of NHI (such as its administration and financing) and their perceptions of the attitudes of colleagues toward NHI, its inevitability, and its anticipated consequences are all related among themselves; and these are related, in turn, with attitudes toward other general and specific aspects of the role of government in health, including Medicare.
- Similarly, attitudes toward different aspects of peer reviews are related, as are the willingness of physicians to delegate different tasks to nonphysicians and their responses to different questions about group practice.

These correlations are the basis for constructing scales for each of these attitude areas, used throughout the book. (For descriptions of these scales, see the section on "Measures and Scales" in the Appendix.) Beyond that, we anticipated correlations *between* the sets of issues, for example, between political and health care issues, to which we turn next.

Attitudes are rarely isolated; rather they form a "system" or "structure" of attitudes (Campbell et al., 1960: 188–215; Converse, 1964).[18] Implicit, if not explicit, in any analysis that sees an object as a system or as a structure is the idea of consistency.[19] But to say that attitudes are structured or related is only a beginning. Questions about that structure that require further analysis include the following:

1. Logically, the strength of the relationships between a set of attitudes, that is, the "tightness" of the structure, may vary from zero, in which case it is inappropriate even to speak of these attitudes as structured, to a situation in which all of the attitudes in a set are very highly correlated, approaching unity.

The tightness of a structure may vary according to such characteristics as the intensity with which the attitudes are held, their salience, the degree to which they are linked to interests and knowledge, and the sophistication of the persons holding these attitudes. Ladd and Lipset note, for example, that "academics are entirely unlike mass publics in that they show a remarkable consistency of ideas across a wide range of issues. Dealing with ideas is their business, and maintaining consistency among them is their special skill" (1975: 198).

2. The degree of *differentiation* among a set of attitudes may vary. All the correlations between a number of attitudes may be exactly the same. This would indicate no differentiation. Or, the correlations between some attitudes may be stronger than those between others. These clusters indicate "subsystems" or "substructures." They are evidence of internal differentiation of the larger structure.

The Strategic Use of the Concept of Attitude Structure

The concept of attitude structure, incorporating both attitudes and cognitions, is used in a number of important ways in our analysis.

First, the correlation of an attitude with other attitudes adds to our understanding of the meaning of that attitude. Such an understanding leads to an appreciation of the resistance of attitudes to change while at the same time suggesting possible levers for change. It has direct implications for policy matters.

Second, in Chapter 4 we refer to attitude structure in formulating hypotheses about how objective background characteristics are related to specific attitudes. For example, we predict that physicians from working-class backgrounds would be more likely than physicians from middle-class backgrounds to be attracted to group practice because working-class people emphasize "autonomy" and "independence" less than do middle-class people.

Third, we rely heavily on the idea of attitude structure in examining the dynamics of attitude change in Chapter 6. We use the idea of structure to argue that the change in the attitudes of physicians toward Medicare was due to the Medicare law rather than to a more general, long-term trend in the ideology of physicians; we use the idea of structure in analyzing the *conditions* of change in the attitudes of individual physicians toward Medicare; and we use it to explain why we expect the change in attitudes toward Medicare to *generalize* to other attitudes.

Findings

We originally thought that the attitudes we have examined would divide into three clusters: a "political-orientation" cluster, a "health-care-organization" cluster, and a "government-in-health-and-medical-care" cluster that straddles the first two.* The correlations in Table 2-1 lend some support to this conceptualization. The political items are correlated among themselves, Pearson r's ranging from .37 to .54 and averaging .44, as are the three government-in-health-and-medical-care scales, Pearson r's ranging from .48 to .58, and averaging .52. The health-care-organization items, however, are less highly correlated, r's ranging from .20 to .33, and averaging .25. Physicians' attitudes toward these health care issues reflected, though less strongly than we expected, the objective relationships between these components of health care, discussed earlier in this chapter.

How these three clusters are related to each other is of particular interest. The government-in-health-and-medical-care items (4, 5, 6) are

---

* The political-orientation cluster would include an economic-welfare liberalism scale, political identification, and political party preference. The government-in-health-and-medical-care cluster would include: a "government-in-health" scale to tap attitudes toward the role of government in nonhealth care areas such as hospital construction, medical education, and biomedical research; a "government-in-medicine" scale to tap the role of government in medical care; and a "national health insurance" scale. The health-care-organization cluster would include the issues of group practice, peer reviews, task delegation, physician reimbursement, and prepayment. The scales or items are described in the section on "Measures and Scales" in the Appendix.

In Chapters 4, 5, and 7 we use a superscale of "political ideology" that is made up of the economic-welfare liberalism scale, political identification, and political party preference. And we use the "government-in-medicine" scale to best represent the general area of the role of government-in-health-and-medical-care.

Table 2-1. Correlations Between Physicians' Attitudes Toward Political and Health Care Issues[a]

	Political Orientation Issues			Gov't in Health and Medical Care Issues			Health Care Organization Issues				
	1	2	3	4	5	6	7	8	9	10	11
	Economic-welfare liberalism	Political identification	Political party preference	Gov't. in health	Gov't. in medicine	NHI	Group practice	Peer reviews	Task delegation	Physician reimbursement	Prepayment
Political Orientation Issues											
1. Economic-welfare liberalism	—	.37	.40	.39	.44	.42	.19	.16	.10	.28	.19
2. Political identification		—	.54	.30	.40	.44	.22	.24	.18	.19	.26
3. Political party preference			—	.29	.36	.42	.18	.15	.10	.23	.24
Gov't in Health and Medical Care Issues											
4. Gov't-in-health				—	.49	.48	.25	.29	.21	.33	.28
5. Gov't-in-medicine					—	.58	.30	.29	.22	.34	.34
6. NHI (National Health Insurance)						—	.41	.32	.26	.49	.44
Health Care Organization Issues											
7. Group practice							—	.32	.25	.33	.25
8. Peer reviews								—	.28	.20	.20
9. Task delegation									—	.20	.22
10. Physician reimbursement (salary, capitation, fixed fees, customary fees)										—	.29
11. Prepayment											—

[a]The figures in the table are Pearson r's.

43

indeed about equally correlated with the political-orientation and health-care-organization issues; the former r's range between .29 and .44, and average .38, while the latter range from .21 to .49, and average .32. The political and the health care issues, by contrast, are only weakly correlated, r's ranging from .10 to .28, and average only .19.

A factor analysis of the eleven attitude measures yields similar results, shown in a different form in Table 2-2. In a principal factor analysis, two-factor solution using varimax rotation (using "PA2" in the SPSS manual—see Nie et al., 1975: 474-6, 480), the three political items load most highly on the first factor (the "political" factor), and only weakly on the second factor (the "health-care-organization" factor). Note that the government-in-health-and-medical-care measures load about equally on both factors. The health-care-organization issues, finally, load on the second factor, but barely on the political factor.

Politicization of Physicians' Attitudes

It is not surprising that the views of physicians about the role of government in health care and other health-related activities, including specific programs like Medicare and NHI, are highly linked to their political thinking. The issue of the proper role of government in health is "similar" to, part-and-parcel of, a general set of issues dealing with the proper role of government in other economic-welfare activities, such as unem-

Table 2-2. Factor Loadings from Varimax, Orthogonal Rotated Factor Matrix

Issues	Factor 1 (political)	Factor 2 (health care)
Political Orientation		
Political party preference	.	.10
Political identification	.64	.21
Economic-welfare liberalism	.55	.24
Gov't in Health and Medical Care		
NHI (National Health Insurance)	.50	.64
Gov't-in-medicine	.50	.49
Gov't-in-health	.39	.46
Health Care Organization		
Prepayment	.25	.43
Physician reimburse	.23	.50
Peer reviews	.14	.45
Group practice	.14	.54
Task delegation	.06	.43

ployment, poverty, housing, education, and the like (see, for example, Campbell et al., 1960: 194–198).

But the politics of physicians also "spill over" to their attitudes toward issues that, on the face of it, would appear to be less "political"—group practice, peer reviews, task delegation, salaried reimbursement, prepayment.[20] The degree to which issues are "politicized" in the thinking of the nation's physicians depends on the extent to which they are topics of political debate and controversy. The rights of physicians in group and salaried practice have been the subjects of intense legislative activity and court decisions in the past ("The American Medical Association: power, purpose, and politics. . . ," 1954: 976–996). In the early seventies, group practice and peer reviews emerged as national issues with the enactment of the HMO and PSRO programs, and questions about physician reimbursement and prepayment were intensified, first because of their inclusion in some NHI plans designed to reform the health care system, and more recently, as mechanisms to control the high cost of health care.[21]

Physicians are not unaware of the connection between politics and the organization of health care. Asked how important "medical care issues" would be in the 1984 national elections, nearly 80 percent responded "very important" (26%) or "fairly important" (53%) (American Medical Association, 1983b: 19).

In a speech about Medicare before the AMA House of Delegates in 1965, however, the newly elected president of the association said:

> If the law [Medicare] works badly, a doctor must call this up to the attention of his patients. On the other hand, the physician *must not let his political philosophy* be the criterion of his judgment as to what constitutes good or inferior quality care. Such judgment must be objective and based on *purely scientific grounds*" (*New York Times*, June 21, 1965, p. 1) (*Emphasis added*)

Clearly our findings undercut appeals by organized medicine to "keep politics out of health."

Summary

Although physicians were more conservative than the general public in their political and health care views, substantial proportions took liberal positions on these issues. The strength of liberal thinking among physicians and the gap between them and the general public varied, of course, from issue to issue and over time. The medical profession is not, as often portrayed, monolithically conservative. There is great diversity:

- Nearly a quarter (23%) identified themselves as "liberal" in their political thinking, and nearly a third (31%) identified with the Democratic party;
- a majority (56%) favored "some form of national health insurance";
- more than half (54%) considered a "small" group practice as most desirable for themselves (assuming "your income . . . were the same"), and a fourth (24%) chose a "large" group; only a fifth chose "solo practice" or a "partnership of two physicians";
- four-fifths (83%) favored peer reviews in hospitals, nearly half (48%), in doctors' offices;
- two-thirds (64%) would use a nurse-practitioner or a physician's assistant in their practice, but they were much more willing to delegate some tasks than others;
- three-fifths (61%) would be agreeable to *fixed fees* under national health insurance, a fourth, to *capitation* (for family doctors), and one out of seven (14%) to *salaried* reimbursement.

Physicians' underestimate of their colleagues' support for national health insurance is a clear instance of "pluralistic ignorance," individuals assuming that they are alone in holding an attitude, not knowing that others privately share it. But why is the medical profession as a whole perceived by both physicians themselves and the general public to be more conservative than it is in fact? We suggested that both groups, lacking other sources of information, attribute to the profession the historically conservative policies of the AMA.

And physicians' attitudes toward health care issues, especially those that involved the direct participation of government in health care, are closely correlated with their political attitudes. Even issues that on the face of them have little to do with political ideology (group practice, peer review, task delegation, physician reimbursement, and prepayment) are "politicized" in the thinking of physicians themselves.

We turn next, in Chapter 3, to describe a profile of the medical profession in terms of the social and professional characteristics of physicians.

Notes

1. The figures in this discussion are drawn from: USDHHS, 1982.

2. Perhaps the most dramatic trend in health care has been the explosion of medical knowledge and technology. Organ transplants, neonatal care units, kidney dialysis, laser surgery, nuclear medicine, and NMR (nuclear magnetic resonance) scanners are among the

discoveries that have revolutionized medicine. In turn, they have raised a host of legal, ethical, and financial questions. A 1976 HEW report observes, "The U.S. health care system has fallen rather blindly in love with sophisticated medical technology" (USDHEW, 1976: 34).

Because many of the new devices and procedures prolong life without providing a cure for disease, these innovations have been labeled "half-way" technologies (Thomas, 1977). Coronary care units provide a vivid example of the institutionalization of new technologies whose effectiveness remains controversial. While advances in neonatal care raise the issue of the viability of the fetus at earlier and earlier stages of development, other ethical and legal dilemmas are raised by the ability of medicine to extend indefinitely the lives of patients whose chances of even partial recovery seem dim.

The diffusion of medical technology is propelled by a number of factors including fee-for-service reimbursement, third-party financing and the role of the "latest" in medical technology in defining the prestige of acute-care hospitals and their ability to attract and retain physicians (Reilly and Legge, 1982). Even more fundamental, however, are the current values of the medical profession and society, which "dictate the most appropriate massive medical intervention permitted by available facilities" regardless of cost or other constraints (Berki, 1983).

3. This trend is only slightly affected by the establishment of family practice as a specialty in the mid-seventies and its growth from 3.1 percent of all physicians in 1975 to 6.4 percent in 1981. A discussion of the implications of specialization trends must be qualified, however, by introducing the concept of "primary care"—"first contact, routine medical treatment, and care coordination" (USDHHS, 1980: 80), to the extent that primary care is provided by specialists, mainly by internists and pediatricians.

4. See Stevens, 1971, for a comprehensive historical account of specialization in American medicine. On the intellectual and social factors spurring specialization in science see Cole and Zuckerman, 1975; in the professions, with particular reference to medicine, see Bucher and Strauss, 1961. Case studies are particularly illuminating. On ophthalmology, see Rosen, 1944; on physical rehabilitation in medicine, see Gritzer, 1978; on pediatrics, Halpern, 1984; on geriatrics, Stevens, 1977, and Colombotos and Indyk, 1983.

5. Figures vary according to different sources because of different definitions of group practice. The current definition used in the latest AMA study is:

> Group medical practice is the application of medical services by three or more physicians formally organized to provide medical care, consultation, diagnosis, and/or treatment through the joint use of equipment and personnel, and with the income from medical practice distributed in accordance with methods previously determined by members of the group. (American Medical Association, 1982a)

6. In 1979 it was estimated that 38 percent of the physicians in the United States (excluding interns and residents) were "mainly" salaried (Physicians Forum, 1982: 11). This estimate, however, was based on assumptions about the proportion of physicians who were "predominantly" on salary in certain activity categories.

7. General analyses of AMA policies appear in: "The American Medical Association: Power, purpose and politics in organized medicine," 1954: 976–1018; Harris, 1966; Rayack, 1967; Stevens, 1971: passim; Tatalovich, 1971; Feldstein, 1977: 27–76; Starr, 1982: passim. Most of these studies are critical of the AMA. For a more sympathetic treatment, including a summary of a rebuttal to charges that AMA policies were obstructive and reactionary, see the recent "authorized history" of the AMA by Campion (1984, particularly pp. 521–529).

8. But the association of science with progressive thinking should not be overdrawn. On the resistance to change in science, see Stern, 1941. Also, Kuhn's notion of "scientific revolution" stresses resistance to new paradigms in science (Kuhn, 1962). A somewhat related, but conceptually distinct, question involves what we might call the "therapeutic conservatism" of medical practitioners. Three-fourths were "more inclined to rely on accepted forms of treatment" rather than "to try out new forms of treatment" (Q.42). But the responses of physicians to this question were unrelated to their political or health care views.

9. See Interview Schedule in Appendix.

10. A somewhat different line of investigation would examine whether different segments of the profession, for example, practitioners and academic physicians, differed among themselves with respect to the acceptability of the activities depending on their salience and meaning. For example, "medical care to poor people" and "where doctors practice" may have a greater impact on practitioners than on academic physicians, whereas "priorities in biomedical research" and "medical school curricula" may have a greater impact on academic physicians.

11. Other studies of the attitudes of physicians toward NHI during the first half of the seventies yielded closely similar results (Strickland, 1972: 68).

Asked about specific features of NHI in our national study, physicians generally favored the more conservative version. They preferred a plan financed by private insurance rather than one financed by employer-employee contributions through social security; they preferred a plan administered by Blue Cross, Blue Shield and by private insurance companies rather than by the federal government; and they preferred a plan that did not support the development of group practice. For a more detailed analysis of our 1973 data on the attitudes of physicians toward these and other components of NHI, see Colombotos, Kirchner, and Millman, 1975b.

12. The tendency to underestimate liberal opinion and overestimate conservative opinion is not limited to "rank-and-file" physicians. In a survey of the AMA House of Delegates, members perceived the House as a whole as more conservative than themselves (The AMA House of Delegates: Does it really speak for American Medicine? 1971: 39). And in a 1979 survey of the American public, two-thirds of those who ventured a guess thought that the AMA opposed any kind of NHI (American Medical Association, 1979).

13. The same pattern was found in a 1955 national study of physicians (National Opinion Research Center, undated).

14. For a fuller discussion of sources of resistance to peer reviews, including an empirical test of the "clinical mentality," see Colombotos, Kirchner, and Millman, 1975a.

15. The absolute levels of agreement with salary, capitation, and fixed fees would probably have been higher if the questions did not refer to payment "under NHI" or if the context were left unspecified. For analyzing relationships between the attitudes of physicians toward method of reimbursement and other factors, however, we would argue that our measures are appropriate.

16. Note that the response alternatives in the question do not clearly specify the presence or absence of a third party; whether the patient is an individual subscriber or a member of a group plan; whether the insurance system is voluntary or compulsory; or whether the third party is a private carrier or government. Each of these attributes is likely to affect the attitudes of physicians toward alternatives.

17. With the exception of Medicare, our comparisons are based on identically worded items in surveys conducted at approximately the same time. For those interested in public opinion data on political, social welfare, and health insurance issues, see especially Schiltz,

1970; Erskine, 1975; also, consult survey archival sources such as those available at the Roper Public Opinion Research Center; Jeffe and Jeffe, 1984). For a rare comparative study of the views on health care issues of members of the public, physicians, physician leaders, and hospital administrators, see Louis Harris and Associates, 1984.

18. There are many different conceptualizations of "attitude." (For a thorough review of attitude research and theory, see McGuire, 1969.) In our view, attitudes have two components: a *cognitive* aspect—an object, person, issue, or idea, and an *affective* aspect—approaching-withdrawing, liking-disliking, favoring-opposing. Thus, we may speak of people's attitudes toward national health insurance, blacks, the equal-rights amendment, or chocolate ice cream. Concepts that involve only a *cognitive* aspect—perceptions, beliefs, expectations, knowledge, and the like—may be empirically related to attitudes toward a given object, say NIH, as we have just noted. We make this analytic distinction between attitudes and cognitions, recognizing that the distinction may be blurred (see, e.g., Hyman, 1955: 97-105).

The "consistency" of attitudes and behavior is a complex question that has engaged the active interest of social psychologists over the years, and we will not go into it here in any detail. Our general position is that to accept the argument that attitudes and behavior are not perfectly consistent is not to say that they are totally unrelated, either. We view attitudes as probability statements about overt behavior in specific social situations. The accuracy of these probability statements depends on a host of factors, including other, perhaps conflicting, attitudes relevant to the behavior in question and the constraints of the immediate social situation. Thus, the question of whether attitudes are or are not consistent with behavior gives way to the more fruitful question of under what *conditions* are attitudes useful as reasonably accurate predictors of specific behavior. (For a good discussion of the issue, see Hill, 1981.)

19. The proposition of a "strain toward consistency" has a long history. In anthropology and sociology it describes relations between elements of culture and society; in psychology, it describes relations between elements of personality, including attitudes. "Consistency," it is postulated, leads to stability in these systems; "inconsistency" leads to change.

On the face of it, the notion of consistency is a simple idea, but this simplicity is deceptive. The criterion for determining *interpersonal* consistency, assuming the persons like each other, is agreement between them in their opinions and attitudes toward a given object or issue. Disagreement leads to change either in the subject's attitude toward the object or toward the other person(s) (Newcomb, 1953).

Intrapersonal consistency is more problematic. What does it mean to say that two or more attitudes are "consistent" or "inconsistent"? McGuire has identified two main criteria (McGuire, 1960: 70-73).

The population parameter (statistical) method is based on the empirical correlation between two or more attitudes. For example, physicians who are politically liberal are more likely than those who are conservative to be in favor of national health insurance. Thus, liberals who favor NHI and conservatives who oppose it are "consistent"; liberals who oppose NHI and conservatives who favor it are "inconsistent." (The term "cross-pressures," which may refer to either attitude or group variables, is based—when used in voting studies—on such empirical correlations [Berelson, Lazarsfeld, and McPhee, 1954; Campbell et al., 1960].)

The formal model method is based on a logical syllogistic relationship between sets of attitudes. For example, politically liberal views and support for national health insurance are consistent *because* support for NHI is *part-and-parcel* of a general perspective that supports the participation and responsibility of government in addressing social problems.

This is a "similarity" relation. Or, opposition to formal peer review programs and opposition to NHI are "consistent" *because* it is generally recognized that government programs like NHI inevitably *lead to* more formalized peer review programs. This is an "instrumentality" relation (McGuire, 1960).

Logical relations between attitudes may, of course, be reflected in *empirical* correlations between them in a population on the assumption that a good part of the population perceives the same "logical" relations between issues as does the observer. In such instances, "psychological" consistency corresponds with "logical" consistency.

It is informative to note how the experimental and survey approaches to the study of attitude change differ in dealing with intrapersonal consistency: (1) Consistency theories by experimental social psychologists have reached a high level of complexity. Degree of inconsistency, awareness of inconsistency and techniques of increasing awareness, effects of temporal factors on awareness of inconsistency, methods of resolving inconsistency—these and other factors have been (or can be) manipulated experimentally. In surveys, the concept of consistency has remained theoretically primitive; the concept is merely asserted. (2) The criterion for determining consistency in experimental studies is often a logical, or psychological, one. In surveys, the criterion is usually statistical (Berelson, Lazarsfeld, and McPhee, 1954); Rosenberg (1957) uses both criteria in his analysis of change in career decisions, without noting the difference.

The two research traditions—the experimental and the survey—have gone separate ways. For example, in the 900-page reader on cognitive consistency, edited by Abelson and others (1968), there is not one reference to a survey.

20. Similar findings have been obtained in other investigations of the attitudes of physicians and residents (Mechanic, 1974; Louis Harris and Associates, 1981: 95).

21. In the New York State study, the strength of the intercorrelations between the political views of physicians and their attitudes toward peer reviews increased steadily after Medicare because, we speculate, of the debate about formal utilization review programs required by Medicare. But issues may also be "politicized" to the extent that groups in society are successful in keeping them *off* the political agenda (see Schattschneider, 1960).

The concept of "medicalization," the conversion of moral, social, or political problems into medical ones, is germane to this discussion. In this context, "demedicalization" may be close cousin to "politicization." (On medicalization and demedicalization in American society, see Fox, 1977.)

3 A Social and Professional Profile of Physicians

In this chapter we describe the objective social background and professional characteristics of physicians. Because every physician fills many positions, or statuses, in society and in the organization of the medical profession, and because "status-sets" and "status-sequences" are patterned rather than random combinations of characteristics (see Merton, 1957: 380–384), we also look at how social and professional characteristics of physicians are related. Finally, we examine trends in the social and professional composition of the profession as reflected in the age differences of our study sample and based on data from other sources.

Interest in the social and professional characteristics of physicians stems from several sources. One is a commitment to eliminating traditional barriers to entry into a high status occupation, such as encountered by women and members of certain ethnic minorities. Another is the concern of health planners with issues of physician maldistribution according to specialty and geographic location. Just as the reasons for policy interest in objective status characteristics of physicians vary, so there are several bases for theoretical interest in such characteristics. This is evident in the many studies describing the social origins of business leaders, civil servants, and professional groups. A few of these studies examine the effects of specific background characteristics on specific attitudes, behavior, and careers (see Chapter 4, notes 3 and 4). Alternatively, such studies examine social origins as indicators of the profession's status or of its actual or potential political power. These alternative orientations are not unrelated.

When status and power are the focal interests, there tends to be an emphasis on theories of social *selection* into professional groups rather than on theories of socialization. By contrast, an emphasis on socialization processes tends to dominate studies that are mainly concerned with a profession's ideological stances. In fact, both socialization and selection processes are needed to account for the attitudes and influence of a profession as a group at any given time.

Within the focus on socialization, alternative theoretical positions are found (discussed in Chapter 4). Notably, there are the contrasting views on whether early or later socialization is the more significant determinant of current attitudes. Theories that favor early socialization point to the impact of shaping previously unformed attitudes and suggest that early attitudes persist or lead to selective learning in subsequent socialization experiences. Other theorists consider that later socialization experiences have greater impact on current attitudes; they argue that recent experiences have greater salience for current situations.

The distinction between social and professional characteristics is linked to theories of socialization over the life cycle. For the most part, social characteristics indicate sources of early or childhood socialization, although some, such as gender and ethnicity, extend throughout life. Professional characteristics refer to adult socialization, including formal and informal learning during professional training and later working arrangements.

Although the distinction between social and professional characteristics is clear in the abstract, certain specific statuses are hard to classify. Income is an example, serving as a status indicator that has its basis in professional activity but that also refers to a measure of social ranking that is not limited to professional participation. Foreign versus American medical education is another ambiguous indicator because it is empirically so closely associated with cultural origins. Over 80 percent of foreign medical graduates in our 1973 national sample were foreign born; more than 90 percent of those born abroad were trained there.

Specifically, in this chapter we examine the following social characteristics—socioeconomic, religious, and racial background, generational status, regional origins, and gender. We also examine the following professional characteristics—worksetting (a typology that includes the main type of activity, i.e., patient care, teaching, administration, or research; the organization of work, whether solo or group; and the method of reimbursement, whether salaried or fee-for-service); specialty; and board certification. Unless indicated otherwise, the data come from our 1973 national sample of senior physicians.

Social Characteristics

Socioeconomic Origins

Are physicians drawn from a wide spectrum of society in terms of their parents' socioeconomic status? We review several measures that bear on this question: the respondents' perception of their parents' social class (Q.92); whether the fathers of respondents were physicians (Q.85A); whether their fathers (other than those who were physicians) were self-employed (Q.85C); their fathers' educational attainment (Q.84);[1] and whether the respondents were in debt when they graduated from medical school (Q.94), as an indicator of family income. Except for debts, all these measures refer to when the respondent was in his or her late adolescence.

To make comparisons with the general population, we use relevant census data for the parents' generation. Obviously the comparison can be only approximate, since the sample ranges in age from about 30 years to over 70 years, with a median age of about 45. We decided that data from the 1940 census would apply best—that is, about 30 years between the median age of physicians when we interviewed them and their teen years.

Social Class Origins

The high prestige of the medical profession in our society confers on all its members a secure place in the upper-middle class. For some, lineage and wealth further enhance this position. Half our study sample perceived themselves as coming from backgrounds described as "upper class" (4%) or "upper-middle" (47%);[2] 29 percent, from "lower-middle-class" backgrounds; and the remaining 18 percent, from "working-class" backgrounds. This means that about half the physicians moved up the social class ladder, some quite sharply. Navarro (1976: 143–145) reports that only 12 percent of the medical students come from families whose income is below the national median, and that this percentage has remained the same since 1920. (See also Gee and Glaser, 1958: 247–248; Lyden, Geiger, and Peterson, 1968.)

Medical Origins

A more specific indication of social class "inheritance" involves choice of a medical career in relation to the father's occupation. If that choice were random, we would expect fewer than 1 percent of the current generation of physicians to have physician-fathers; instead, we found 14 percent. There are few data that permit us to compare this result with earlier periods in medicine, or with other occupations. A small-scale study of birth cohorts of physicians from 1870–1920, which sampled two cities in Massachusetts and two in Ohio, found a decline of those with physician-fathers from 22 percent in the oldest cohort to 9 percent in the youngest (Adams, 1953: 407).

A 1953 study of entrants to the medical school and to the law school at one university found no notable difference in the percentages who had a parent in the same profession as their choice—17 percent of medical students and 15 percent of law students (Thielens, 1957: 137).

Self-Employed Fathers

The issue of salaried practice, raised in Chapter 2, led us to query whether the fathers of physicians had been in salaried employment or had, instead, been self-employed. About half of the respondents' fathers were self-employed, more than double the figure we would expect to find in the general population, since about a fifth of employed males in the fathers' generation were self-employed. The finding suggests that the characteristic emphasis by physicians on autonomy in their work may have its source in—or be sustained by—early childhood experience.

Fathers' Education

Only about one-quarter of the respondents came from families in which their father had gone beyond the baccalaureate level in formal education, and a nearly equal percentage came from families where the father had no more than eight years of schooling. Thus most respondents have attained a higher educational status than their fathers, often much higher.

Nevertheless, compared to the general population, physicians are drawn disproportionately from the more highly educated segment. Whereas, in 1940, only 5 percent of adult males had graduated from college, 37 percent of the physicians' fathers had college degrees; conversely, 76 percent of adult males in the general population in 1940 had not graduated from high school, compared to only 32 percent of physicians' fathers (U.S. Bureau of the Census, 1982: 143).

Debts at Graduation from Medical School

Whether one is in debt upon graduation from medical school is at best a weak indicator of parental family income (especially since the question included "debts to your family that you felt obliged to pay back"). Whether debts are incurred is also a function of the varying costs of medical education, the availability of loans, and individual and family norms about a young adult's responsibility for the costs of his/her professional education. Nevertheless, the finding that nearly half (46%) of the senior physicians were in debt when they graduated is consistent with the similar number whose perceived social origin was "lower middle," "working," or "lower" class.

More directly, of course, the presence of debts indicates financial pressures on the young physician which may limit the amount of postgraduate training he or she chooses to undertake, and also may affect the type of activity and/or the form of practice selected.

The evidence we have reviewed supports the general perception that physicians are disproportionately drawn from high socioeconomic backgrounds. Nevertheless there was considerable variation, with one-fifth to one-quarter found to have grown up in rather humble circumstances, as measured by the education of their fathers or by their own perception of their parents' social class.

Ethnic-Cultural Origins

Ethnic groupings within American society have several, partially overlapping bases: national origin, race, and religion. Ethnicity and social class are strongly associated in the general population, with nonwhite and/or non-English-speaking ethnic minorities overrepresented in lower-class strata. Consequently, these ethnic minorities are generally underrepresented among physicians, with some exceptions, as described below.

Generational Status

As noted above, we classified respondents according to whether they were born abroad (first-generation Americans), or born in the United States with one or both parents having been born abroad (second-generation Americans), or both parents and the self born in the United States (third-plus generation Americans). By far most of the foreign-born physicians came to the United States after graduating from medical school, and nearly all the physicians born in the United States attended medical school in this country. The categories "foreign-born" (i.e., "first-generation") and Foreign Medical Graduate (FMG) are practically coterminous (Colombotos, Charles, and Kirchner, 1977: 604). Thus it was not possible, in this study, to separate statistically the influence of early national cultural origins and of the country of professional training on the attitudes of physicians toward political and health care issues. In 1973, 13 percent of the senior physicians had received their medical training abroad. In recent years the number and proportion of those physicians among the FMG's who were born in the United States has been increasing (Mick and Worobey, 1984: 701–702).

In terms of generational status, a much larger percentage had childhood exposure to foreign culture: in addition to the 13 percent of the physicians who were foreign born, nearly a fourth (25%) were born in the United States, with one or both parents born abroad. Together, these two groups (first- and second-generation Americans) make up fully two-fifths of the medical profession. These figures far exceed the proportions of comparable subgroups in the general U.S. population. In 1970, only 5 percent of the total population was foreign born; and only 12 percent of the total population was native born, with one or both parents born abroad (U.S. Bureau of the Census, 1982: 36).

Why the excess proportion of persons of foreign extraction among physicians compared to the rest of the population?[3] The explanations probably differ for first-generation and for second-generation groups.

For the foreign born, one has to consider both "push" and "pull" factors that might account for the high proportion of professionals, specifically physicians, among immigrants. These factors include political, economic, and professional situations both in the country of origin and in the United States (Colombotos, Charles, and Kirchner, 1977; Foster, 1976). Historical events in different parts of the world are reflected in the national composition of different age groups of immigrant physicians. Older immigrant physicians (like older nonphysician immigrants) came mainly from central and eastern Europe. Most of them migrated in the 1930s and 1940s. Younger physician immigrants, especially those who are now working here as housestaff, are also more recent migrants. They come predominantly from Asia or the Philippines and other "third-world" or "developing" countries (Sun Valley Forum, 1975). The immigration laws of the United States have also changed over the years, at some periods favoring certain nationalities; they have also varied, sometimes encouraging and at other times discouraging the entry of professional/technical personnel, specifically physicians.[4]

Apart from specific push-and-pull factors, a more general theoretical explanation for the higher proportion of first-generation physicians than first-generation Americans in the general population can be derived from the proposition that the professions, particularly those that are scientifically based, tend toward internationalism, as one expression of the more basic value orientation of "universalism" (Hughes, 1971: 386).

The explanation for the relatively high proportion of second-generation Americans among physicians, compared to the rest of the population, introduces other factors. The parents of this group must have migrated predominantly in the 20-year period between 1920 and 1940, and therefore their cultural origins are mainly central and eastern European. The assimilation of members from this group into American society—in spite of their generally humble social class origins and continued low status in this country—apparently rests on strong parental support for their children and on high aspirations for them to enter high-status occupations (Glazer and Moynihan, 1963).

Religious Origins

Religious and national origins are closely associated. A high proportion of older first-generation physicians and of second-generation physicians (the groups that stem from central and eastern Europe) have Jewish backgrounds, whereas the younger first-generation physicians are more likely to have Catholic or non-Christian (Hindu, Moslem, or other) backgrounds. Third-plus-generation Americans are most likely to have Protestant origins.

Prior research has documented the predilection among Jews in the United States for their sons to enter medicine, consistent with the more general "passion for education" among Jews (Greeley, 1963: 161; Glazer and Moynihan, 1963: 156–157; Davis, 1965). Of course, the desire had to be matched by the opportunity. Specifically, the issue is whether anti-Semitism limited access to medical education for physicians active in the profession in 1973. Even a speculative answer is complicated. Open anti-Semitism in pre-World War II Europe may have contributed to the high proportion of Jews among immigrant and second-generation physicians. As for medical education in the United States, Glazer and Moynihan (1963: 156–157) concluded that by the 1960s "qualified Jewish students have no problem getting into a medical school," in part because of the founding of Einstein Medical College, which welcomes Jewish students.[5]

Eighteen percent of the physicians were brought up Jewish (Q.81); this compares to 3 percent of the nation's population reported to be Jewish in a Bureau of the Census study in 1957. Fifty-one percent of the physician sample reported Protestant origins, compared to 66 percent of the nation's population in 1957. There was little or no difference between the physician sample and the 1957 population of the United States in percentages reported as Catholics (23 and 26%, respectively), "other religions" (5 and 1%) or "no religion" (3% in each).

Thus, if we consider religious origins, Jews are overrepresented and Protestants underrepresented among physicians relative to the general population. There is little difference in the picture when we consider present religious affiliation (Q.82), except that notably more physicians report no affiliation in the present (15%) than in their background (5%). This shift does not seem to reflect a general population trend, since a 1973 Roper sample of the U.S. population 18 years and older found only 1 percent who reported "no religion," the same as in the 1957 Bureau of Census sample. To balance the implication that medical training generally conflicts with religious orientation, we should note that in answer to a question on religiosity, over 70 percent of the sample considered themselves either "moderately religious" (57%) or "deeply religious" (14%); most of the remainder were "largely indifferent to religion" (26%) rather than "basically opposed to religion" (3%).

Unless otherwise noted, we use the measure of religious background in our subsequent analyses rather than current affiliation or religiosity. This emphasis is in keeping with our interest in the effect of early social origins on the current attitudes of physicians.

Race[6]

Whites make up an overwhelmingly large majority of the profession, in fact, a majority that is disproportionately large relative to the general population. Compared to 93 percent of the physicians who were white, the 1970 census estimated that 89 percent of the population in the United States 25 years or older were white, 9 percent black, and 1.5 percent, other nonwhite (U.S. Bureau of the Census, 1982: 27).

More detailed figures suggest more clearly the disadvantage of American blacks in terms of entering the medical profession. Most of the nonwhite physicians were foreign born and trained, and the majority of them were orientals, followed by "other races," mainly East Indians. Blacks born in the United States were one-third of all nonwhite physicians, making up only 2 percent of the physicians born in the United States.

The legacy of racial discrimination in the larger society accounts, in part, for these figures. In 1970, only 4 percent of adults who had completed college were nonwhite. Many of those blacks attended predominantly black colleges, which have poorer educational resources, particularly in the science fields required for entry into medicine. There is no question that active racial discrimination prevailed in the American medical profession. Although many medical schools are now making conscious efforts to counteract this historical pattern,[7] the possibility of informal discrimination persists.

Institutional responses to the earlier segregation of nonwhite physicians also persists. Two medical schools—Meharry Medical College in Tennessee and Howard University in Washington, D.C.—and one medical association—the National Medical Association (NMA)—predominantly serve nonwhite students and physicians. The latter was formed to provide a professional association for blacks who used to be excluded from local medical societies and from the American Medical Association.

U.S. Regional Origins

It is widely assumed that regional cultural differences in the United States are declining. Glenn and Simmons (1967), however, examined national opinion data for the 1950s and concluded that, on the contrary, regional differences on a wide range of attitudes were increasing. The differences were larger for younger than older groups. South versus non-South contrasts were the largest, but differences were also apparent in other pairings of four standard groupings of states into regions: Northeast, North Central, West, and South.

It is interesting that most physicians lived in the same region, even the same state, in 1973 as they did before attending medical school (Q.80). Thirty-three percent grew up in the Northeast; 29 percent, North Central; 26 percent, South; and 12 percent, West. When this distribution was compared with the U.S. population in 1940, the small differences that were found suggest that the Northeast "overproduced" and the South "underproduced" physicians, while the other two regions are proportionately represented among physicians.[8]

Gender

The sex-typing of occupations is a widespread phenomenon. Medicine is a prime example, with maleness as a powerful "latent identity" even though women have earned medical degrees in the United States since the nineteenth century.

The proportion of American physicians who are women actually has fluctuated notably over the decades since that date. It was higher in the early 1900s when there was no legal protection against discrimination than in the early 1970s, some years after such protection had been federally enacted. In 1973, only 5 percent of our senior physician sample were women.

In spite of many signs of legal prohibitions against sex discrimination and institutional acceptance of women in medicine, including a rapidly rising percentage of women among recent entrants, observers have documented the persistence of informal discrimination.

Women physicians, like black physicians, founded their own professional association—the American Medical Women's Association (AMWA)—in response to early exclusion from local medical societies and the AMA. AMWA persists although women now participate in the full range of medical organizations.[9]

Professional Characteristics

Next, we turn to differences that derive from the organization of the profession itself; more precisely, these differences express the organization of the profession. They refer to distinctive aspects of the conditions and/or the content of the physicians' work.

Worksetting

Our preliminary analyses revealed clear patterning in the associations among physicians' *main activity* (patient care, teaching, research, or administration), *organization of work* (solo, partnership, group, or large organization), and *method of reimbursement* (proportion of income derived from salary rather than fee-for-service). Based on these patterns, we created a typology—"worksetting"—for subsequent analysis (see "Measures and Scales" in Appendix). The largest category (37%) consists of those whose main activity was patient care and who practiced in a fee-for-service solo or partnership setting. Next, 30 percent were practitioners in group practice, including those who were hospital-based and who were also reimbursed on a fee-for-service basis. A much smaller but still substantial category (18%) consists of those in salaried patient care in group or hospital-based settings. Finally, 16 percent were "nonpractitioners," that is, they spent most of their time in research, teaching, and/or administration and were mainly salaried. About half of this last group included "mixed types" who reported substantial—though secondary—involvement in patient care and who drew income from fee-for-service as well as from salary.

It should be emphasized that although these categories are distinctive in many ways, the typology covers a great deal of diversity in each physician's usual activities and worksettings. Respondents were asked in detail about all their activities, and they were then classified according to the *main* activity in terms of the percentage of time spent in a typical week; this approach revealed that nearly all engaged in some *combination* of patient care with administration, research, and/or training. A third (35%) of all physicians, for example, indicated that they were "currently on the faculty of a medical school."

Those who were mainly nonpractitioners were most likely to be regularly engaged in all of the activity categories. Similarly, most physicians worked in two or more organizational settings during their typical work week. There was less overlap in the method of reimbursement. Only one-third drew income both from salary and fee-for-service; more relied entirely on fee-for-service (37%) than entirely on salary (30%), but the difference between them is not large.

Recognizing that such diversity underlies the worksettings adds interest to our investigation of whether these professional characteristics are related to attitudes on health care issues. Are there clear-cut attitudinal differences among physicians according to their *dominant* worksetting activity? Or do physicians tend to share views because most of them spend at least small portions of their time in several of the worksettings?

Specialty and Board Certification

Much more attention has been paid in the literature to differentiating among physicians according to their specialty than according to their worksetting (see our discussion in Chapters 2 and 4).

Board certification in a specialty is increasingly becoming the standard, although physicians may still choose to identify themselves as a specialist simply by limiting the nature of their practice. Close to half (48%) of our 1973 senior physician sample had attained board certification.

Relationships Among Social and Professional Characteristics

It is in the nature of subcultural differentiation that status characteristics, such as those we have taken up sequentially, are not randomly distributed in relation to each other. In the sociological literature, the processes by which the clustering of statuses occurs have been studied under the headings of status-sets and status-sequences. As study after study shows, even in our open society with its ideals of individual achievement and group assimilation, the distinctive clustering of ascribed and achieved attributes tends to persist over long periods. This is a more technical way of restating Glazer and Moynihan's conclusion from a study of immigrant groups in New York: "the point about the melting pot . . . is that it did not happen" (1963).

We examine status-sets among the medical profession by first considering clusters among social characteristics, then clusters among the professional characteristics, and finally, clusters among social and professional characteristics.

Relationships Among Social Characteristics

The most distinctive patterning observed among physicians is the linkage of foreign birth, race, and religion—in other words, the complex of variables that define ethnic subgroups in the larger society. As in the larger society, but probably more pronounced among physicians, we find distinctive subgroups among those who are foreign born, which reflect changes in the immigration laws. Among the senior physicians, about 25 percent of those who were foreign born are nonwhite; among foreign-born housestaff, 64 percent are nonwhite. Very few of the nonwhite foreign-born physicians are black (ca. 1%); most are oriental or "other" (mainly East Indian). Among physicians born in the United States, fully 97 percent were white.

Differences in religious background are strongly associated with world region of origin: Buddhists, Moslems, and Hindus predominate among physician immigrants from the eastern hemisphere; Catholics predominate among foreign-born physicians from South America and Europe; and Protestants predominate among U.S.-born physicians, especially among blacks. Among both those who were born in the United States and those who were not, Jews make up about 18 percent.

We also find that foreign-born physicians are concentrated geographically in the Northeast, especially in large urban centers. This pattern also applies to the ethnic groups to which they belong, although it is probably accentuated among physicians, since they are more heavily clustered in urban centers than is the general population.

Attesting to the persistence of ethnic groups in the larger society, we find strong linkages of religious background and current geographic location with *parents'* birthplace, when we consider only physicians who themselves were born in the United States. Only 9 percent of the U.S.-born Protestant physicians had a foreign-born parent compared to fully 68 percent of the Jewish U.S.-born physicians; among U.S.-born Catholic physicians, 37 percent have at least one immigrant parent. Second-generation physicians are also more likely to have been brought up and to reside currently in the urbanized regions of the Northeast than are those whose parents were both born in the United States.

Other patterns emerge in relation to foreign origin which are weaker than those covered thus far. They are of particular interest because they presumably do not apply to the larger ethnic groups. First, we find that the proportion of women is higher among foreign-born than among U.S.-born physicians (13% vs. 6%); second, a higher proportion of foreign-born physicians than U.S.-born physicians report upper-class or upper-middle-class parental origins (64% vs. 50%).

In general, we find women were more likely than men to report higher socioeconomic origins (upper-class or upper-middle-class). While the pattern is not strong (65% of women vs. 51% of men), it suggests the underlying socialization and selection processes that account for the under-representation of women in medicine. Financial and motivational obstacles that limit the selection of a medical career for men from lower-class backgrounds are intensified for women. In spite of radical changes in attitudes toward women's work and in the rates of women's participation in paid employment, the cultural norm still places the burden of fulfilling the economic and status needs of the family primarily upon men. This general expectation has different consequences for women from families with greater economic resources than for those from families with fewer. Families that have greater resources can and will assist a daughter, even if they are not enthusiastic about her career plans. Adams and Meidam (1968: 238) found that "the sex ratio, or the number of males in a given [family] size, is related to college attendance only in the case of blue-collar females, with each additional male sibling appearing to lessen her chances of attending college."

Economic obstacles for lower-class aspirants to a medical career are greater for women also because of greater reluctance to acquire debts ("negative dowry"), and a similar reluctance by medical schools to permit women "to incur as much 'credit buying' as men because they would have less opportunity to pay it back" (*The Fuller Utilization of the Woman Physician*, 1968: 65).

Socioeconomic background is also associated, though not strongly, with the religious group origins of physicians. Protestants and those from "other" religions had the greatest proportions of upper- or upper-middle class parents. The former reflects the generally higher social status of Protestants in this country; the latter, made up mostly of foreign-born physicians from the eastern hemisphere, reflects the greater degree of class inheritance of occupations in those cultures.

Catholic physicians, by contrast, were more likely, but only slightly, to report that their parents were lower or working class (24%) than were Protestants, Jews, or those of other religious backgrounds (17–14%).

Although the relationship between race and social class in the United States can be observed in our data, it is attenuated compared to its strength in the larger society: 39 percent of black physicians reported their parents were upper or upper-middle class, compared to 52 percent of white physicians.

In general, the relationships among social background variables are not as strong as those found among several of the professional characteristics examined. This was foreshadowed when we discussed the classification of the sample according to "worksetting."

Relationships Among Professional Characteristics

Interestingly, physicians who do not specialize—general practitioners and family practitioners (GP/FPs)—form the most distinctive "specialty" in terms of the characteristics under review. They were most likely to be in solo or partnership practice (59%), followed by general surgeons with 46 percent. Very few GP/FPs were board-certified (only 9%); psychiatrists were next at a sharply higher level (41%) and the figure ranges upward to a high of 71 percent among surgical subspecialists. In fact, board certification was not even an available option for "general practitioners" until 1975, when the new designation "family practitioner" emerged along with the creation of a corresponding specialty board.

Although GP/FPs were least likely to derive any of their income from salary (58% reported no income from salary followed by 46% of general surgeons), their income was similar to the overall average. How did the specialty groups compare in the other worksettings? Psychiatrists had the highest percentage in salaried patient care (33%), followed by radiologists, anesthesiologists, and pathologists, with 22 percent as a group. The lowest percentage in patient care was the heterogeneous group "all other specialties." That group had the highest proportion who are mainly involved in teaching, administration, or research (49%), followed by 27 percent of internal medicine subspecialists such as cardiologists and pulmonary specialists. This is not surprising when we consider that the former group is made up of specialties that have been created precisely in recognition of emerging nonpatient care roles for physicians in public health, occupational medicine, administrative medicine, and the like.

Considering the remaining worksetting—*fee-for-service* group or hospital-based patient care—the most heavily involved specialties are the grouping of radiologists-anesthesiologists-pathologists (47%) and the grouping of surgical specialists (41%); the lowest percentages in this form of practice are psychiatrists (13%) and "all other specialties" (14%).

Income levels varied with specialty, board certification, and worksetting. Surgeons (general and subspecialty) were most likely to be in the upper income grouping, contrasting sharply with pediatricians and "all other specialties." Those who were board-certified were much more likely than those not board-certified to be in the high income group. Fee-for-service patient care in group or hospital-based practice was the most lucrative of the worksetting categories, contrasting most sharply with those in nonpatient care activities, especially those who were primarily in research.

Relationships Between Social and Professional Characteristics

Considerable interest lies in the linkages between the social background characteristics of physicians and their professional activities and related characteristics. Do the same social statuses that have a powerful influence on individuals' choice of, or acceptance into, a medical career, seem to influence their location within the profession? The answer, as one would expect, is not simple. Some background factors have no noticeable relationship to current professional status, while others do. The latter have received research attention, in part to guide policy on the admission and training of specific social groups in medicine (e.g., women, ethnic minorities, foreign-born-and-trained persons). Other research has examined these relationships from a theoretical perspective using medicine, other practicing professions, and the basic sciences as study sites. The starting point for policy-related research generally is concern about filling "shortages," geographic or specialty; this orientation tends to view the persistence of background influences positively. That is, it suggests that choices of practice setting or specialty that are influenced by one's social status are choices based on a strong commitment. By contrast, theoretically oriented research in scientific professions takes as its starting point the ideal norm that status rewards should be based on performance criteria only. From that point of view, background characteristics are "functionally irrelevant statuses," and evidence of their effects on location in the professional structure is viewed negatively, that is, as undermining the stated goals of the professional enterprise (Cole and Cole, 1973).

Socioeconomic Background

Physicians from lower socioeconomic backgrounds were more likely than those from upper socioeconomic backgrounds to be in general/family practice (see also Kandel, 1960; Lyden, Geiger, and Peterson, 1968). Socioeconomic background had no relationship to physicians' attainment of board certification, worksetting, or amount of professional income. However, when we examined the specific subgroup who had physician-fathers compared to all others, an intriguing, though weak, pattern emerged in relation to specialty. Nearly one-fourth (23%) of general surgeons had physician-fathers compared to only one-tenth (10%) of pediatricians. Indeed, when the specialties are rank-ordered in terms of the percentage of individuals who come from medical families, the order closely corresponds to what physicians perceive as the relative prestige of specialties (Reader, 1958: 177; Schwartzbaum and McGrath, 1972; Shortell, 1974). Surgery is highest in prestige and also in the percentage whose fathers were physicians, while pediatrics, psychiatry, and "all other specialties" are low on both counts.

By comparison with the weak effects of socioeconomic background, gender was clearly related to the patterning of medical careers.

Gender

The main gender differences involved income, both its level and the percentage from salary. Women were more likely than men to be salaried, but the gap in the percentage of women and men who were *fully* salaried (48% vs. 30%) in itself is not enough to account for the large income difference: less than one-third of the men (29%) reported an annual net professional income under $30,000, compared with two-thirds (66%) of the women.

Other data in our study show that women averaged fewer weekly work hours than men, although there was wide variation in work hours among both sexes, and a great deal of overlap between them. Furthermore, as we shall describe presently, women and men differ, though not greatly, in specialty and worksetting distributions; finally, women were slightly less likely than men to be board-certified (35% vs. 49%).

Kehrer's (1976) multivariate analysis of the AMA's 1973 survey of office-based practitioners shows that, even taken together, these characteristics, as well as others (e.g., location of practice) to indicate community income level and demand for service, do not fully account for the sex differential in income. The implication that women experience discrimination in salary levels, or that they have difficulty in attracting patients at levels of fees comparable to those of men, remains in question.

There has been a good deal of speculation and some systematic research on the factors that account for the sex difference in specialty distribution (Grenell, 1980; Lorber, 1984). Traditional sex-role socialization, which emphasizes women's involvement in child care and in the social-emotional needs of others, seems to account for the "overselection" of pediatrics and psychiatry by women. We must emphasize that the percentage differences are not large—for example, 5 percent of men are in pediatrics compared to 16 percent of women; 8 percent of men are in psychiatry compared to 13 percent of women. Women were slightly less likely than men to be in general/family practice (13% vs. 21%) and considerably less likely to be in the surgical specialties (11% vs. 29%). In any case, even pediatrics is not a "woman's specialty," since the great majority of pediatricians are men.

But quite different explanations must be drawn upon to explain women's overrepresentation in the specialties that have been identified as those for "physicians without patients"—radiology, anesthesiology, and pathology. In those specialties, and in the category of "miscellaneous" specialties, the factors usually cited to account for the overrepresentation of women are (1) the possibility of maintaining regular hours, and (2) less need to develop a personal following among patients. Studies have documented the prejudices of patients against seeking treatment from women physicians. Although there may be a change in recent years, there is no recent evidence on this question.

Considering type of activity, women are slightly more likely than men to be in nonpatient care activities. This is difficult to discern because the nonpatient care component of the profession is so small. As we have already suggested, the main difference is in the organizational type of practice among those who are in patient care. Women are less likely than men to be in solo fee-for-service practice (22% vs. 37%). This difference might be attributed to the "entrepreneurial" aspect of private practice; the role of entrepreneur has traditionally been a masculine one in our culture. Another possible factor is the aforementioned problem of building a practice because of the prejudices of patients. And finally, private practice may conflict more with the family obligations of married women.

Religion, Foreign Origin, and Race

Keeping in mind that religion, foreign origin, and race are closely related, we review how each of these background characteristics is related to professional characteristics.

RELIGIOUS BACKGROUND. With the exception of specialty, we find almost no difference in the professional characteristics of Protestant, Catholic, and Jewish physicians in the United States.[10] The religious composition of certain specialties, however, varies considerably. Physicians with Jewish origins make up only 10 or 11 percent of GP/FP's and of general surgeons, but they are fully one-third of psychiatrists.

Protestants constitute the plurality in all specialists, but the range is from 60 percent of general practitioners/family practitioners, to only 38 percent of psychiatrists, and 40 percent of medical subspecialists. The variation among specialists in the percentage who are Catholic is smaller, ranging from about 18 percent of pediatricians and internists, to 31 percent of radiologists-anesthesiologists-pathologists.

There are no notable differences according to religious background in type of professional activity and worksetting, level and source of income, or board certification.

FOREIGN ORIGINS. The professional characteristics of physicians of foreign origin differ in several respects from those who are native-born Americans. As with race, and linked to race, the main difference is in level of income and use of salary as a payment mechanism.

The foreign origin of the parents does not appear to influence the professional career patterns of sons or daughters raised in the United States. Therefore we combine second-generation and third-plus-generation in our discussion for comparison with immigrant physicians, nearly all of whom, it may be recalled, are also foreign trained (FMG's).

We noted earlier that, except for their socioeconomic origins, foreign physicians were more likely than American-born physicians to have lower-status social characteristics: they were more likely to be women, nonwhite, and non-Protestant. Foreign physicians were also more likely than those raised in the United States to be in lower-status specialties, such as pathology, anesthesiology, and psychiatry and to work in salaried practice, and to be less likely to be board-certified. Finally, FMG's earn lower average incomes than USMG's. All of these characteristics compound the social disadvantages stemming from the fact of being foreign-born.

RACE. As we found with the effect of gender, the most glaring difference in professional characteristics among the racial groupings has to do with income—both level of income and the proportion of income that is derived from salary. Only 30 percent of white physicians report incomes of under $30,000, compared to 38 percent of black physicians, 42 percent of oriental physicians, and 56 percent of "other races."[11]

Salary as a source of income also differs notably among the racial groups. The salary pattern, however, does not completely match the income distribution. White physicians are most likely to receive no salary (40%) and are least likely to be fully salaried. This ranking corresponds neatly to the relative standing of whites on income compared to that of the other groups. But the correspondence does not hold when we look at the position of blacks on the two variables: the amount of income and the form of income. Blacks are lowest, as we have seen, in the percentage with high income; but they are next-to-lowest in the percentage who are fully salaried (30%). To complete the picture, orientals have the second-highest proportion who are fully salaried (44%) and "other races" by far the highest (56%).

Because payment mechanism is part of our definition of worksetting, these data anticipate the worksetting differences among the racial groups. Nevertheless, there are further points to be made about the race and worksetting of physicians.

Because salaried payment is characteristic of nonpatient care activities, we might expect that the nonwhite groups are overrepresented in those categories, but that is not the case. The differences, perforce, are small, because the total number in the "pure" nonpatient care categories is small to start with. We find that 7 percent of white physicians are in the combined categories of administration, research, and teaching, compared to 4 percent of blacks, 4 percent of orientals, and none (in our sample) of "other races."

Therefore, the large difference we have found in reliance on salary is due to differences in the arrangements under which patient care is provided: only 16 percent of whites are in salaried patient care compared to 41 percent of "other races," while blacks and orientals are in between. Solo, fee-for-service, practice is most common among blacks (42%) and least common among orientals (23%), changing the ordering of the racial groups that we have reported above. Blacks and "other races" are less likely to be in fee-for-service *group* practice (15% and 16%, respectively) than whites and orientals (30% and 29%, respectively).

Blacks are more likely than the other racial groups to be in General Practice/Family Practice (35% of blacks vs. 24%, 21%, and 11% of "other races," whites, and orientals, respectively). This rank-ordering does not correspond, as one might have expected, to the order of racial groupings according to the percentage who are board-certified: "other races" are least likely to be board-certified (22%), followed by blacks (33%), orientals (40%), and whites (49%).

Considering again specialty, blacks are slightly more likely than the other groups to be in internal medicine (21%) compared to 10 to 14 percent of whites, "other races," and orientals.

Looking at the main primary care specialists, internists and general practitioners, together, we note that 56 percent of black physicians are in those fields, compared to 35 percent of whites and of "other races," and 25 percent of oriental physicians.

Trends

In Chapter 2 we described the major trends in the organization of health care. Some of these trends are reflected in differences in the professional composition of different age groups of our senior physician sample in 1973. Specifically, younger physicians were much more likely than older physicians:

- to be in some form of group or hospital-based practice (68% of those under 35 years of age compared with 25% of those 65 or over);
- to be mainly salaried (55% of those under 35 years of age compared with 20% of those 65 or over); and
- to be in a specialty practice (81% of those under 35 years of age compared with 61% of those 65 or over).[12]

Since the early seventies the trends toward group-based and salaried practice have continued to grow, as we noted in Chapter 2. The trend toward specialization, however, has flattened out. Moreover, the number and proportion of physicians in the "primary care" specialties, notably internal medicine, pediatrics, and family practice (boarded in 1975) have increased significantly in the past decade (USDHHS, 1980: 80; American Medical Association, 1983a: 18).

The influx of FMG's, especially, has declined steadily and sharply since the early 1970s; they constituted nearly half (46%) of all initial licenses in 1972, but only 17 percent by 1981 (Mick and Worobey, 1984: 699).

Age differences in our 1973 physician sample reflect little change in the social composition of the profession up to that time, with one exception:

although the proportion of *first*-generation Americans was remarkably similar in all the age groups (about 10%–15%), the proportion of *second*-generation Americans "dropped" from nearly two-fifths (37%) among those 65 or over to one-in-seven (16%) among those under 35, with a consequent increase in the proportion of third-or-more-generation physicians.

Beyond that, however, there was little change. There was little fluctuation in the socioeconomic background of physicians (beyond small differences in their fathers' education, which is probably explained by secular changes in the level of education in the population), and little in racial and religious background, except for a slight increase in oriental and non-Judeo-Christians among younger physicians. It was too early to assess the impact of the policies of the sixties, which stressed the recruitment of women and minorities.

The sharpest impact on the social composition of the profession in the years ahead will be the increasing influx of women since the sixties. In 1959–60, women made up 6 percent of the freshman class of medical students; in 1970–71, 11 percent; in 1974–75, 22 percent; in 1982–83, 32 percent. Women comprised 6 percent of all physicians (including housestaff) in 1963; 12 percent in 1981 ("Medical education in the United States, 1975–76," 1976: 2962; "Medical Education in the United States, 1982–83," 1983: 1513; American Medical Association, 1983a: 18). If the present rate of recruitment continues, women will make up a fifth of the profession within a few decades.

The recruitment of minority students (blacks, American Indians, Mexican-Americans, and Puerto Ricans in the U.S. mainland) into medical schools has not progressed as rapidly. It rose to an all-time high of 9.7 percent of all students in 1970, where it remained until 1978, after the Bakke decision (Gapen, 1979: 20). By 1982–83, it was barely over 8 percent. The proportion of blacks was 5.7 percent ("Medical education in the United States, 1982–83," 1983: 1513).[13]

There is little evidence of any significant change in the socioeconomic backgrounds of American physicians since the seventies—or, for that matter, over the past half-century. As we noted earlier in this chapter, between 1920 and the early seventies, the proportion of medical students who came from families with an income above the national median remained remarkably stable—nearly 90 percent. In 1981–82, it was about the same ("Parental income of 1981 first-year medical applicants . . . ," 1983). Also, the proportion of physicians with physician-fathers, based on a number of different studies of different populations and samples over the years, has remained remarkably stable—between 12 and 17 percent, with no discernible trend (Thielens, 1957: 137; Gee and Glaser, 1958: 247; Lyden, Geiger, and Peterson, 1968: 57; and our national study in 1973).

A Concluding Note

In Chapter 2 we stressed the diversity of physicians' attitudes toward political and health care issues. In the present chapter, the medical profession emerges as equally diverse in its social background and professional characteristics. How are physicians' attitudes and social and professional characteristics linked? We turn to this question next.

Notes

1. Were we to redo the study, we would also ask about the education and occupation of the respondent's *mother*.

2. This measure of "perceived social class origin" was strongly related to the father's education. Moreover, both correlated highly with a score based on the average levels of education and income for males in these occupations (described in U.S. Bureau of the Census, 1963: 4) in our New York State study sample. See Colombotos (1969d: 21) for a description of the measure of socioeconomic background used in that study and for some methodological notes on the problem.

3. The differences would be reduced only slightly if we were able to compare the physician population with the *adult* population in the United States, which would be technically more appropriate.

4. From 1920 through 1968, quotas were officially based on national origin regardless of occupation. Laws passed in 1965, taking force in 1968, gave preference to occupations designated as in short supply in the United States and/or as highly trained. These criteria favored physicians. New laws were passed in 1973 placing restraints on the entry of foreign medical graduates (Mick and Worobey, 1981); these of course did not affect the composition of our sample.

5. As the Coles have pointed out in detail in their study of discrimination in the sciences (1973, 1979), data on the proportionate or disproportionate representation of a group in an occupation reveal little or nothing by themselves about whether the group has encountered discrimination. One needs to know the relative numbers and qualifications of applicants. The Coles's major interest is in whether discrimination occurs *within* the sciences, (i.e., whether it affects those who have completed the relevant education). Hall's early study of sponsorship patterns affecting the careers of medical practitioners in a single community (1948) also deals with discrimination on the basis of religion and national origin among those in the profession rather than with the question of opportunity to become physicians.

6. We include a section here on the racial background of American physicians even though we do not examine the relationship between race and attitudes in Chapter 4. Such an analysis would be quite limited statistically because of the small number of nonwhite physicians. We have found elsewhere, however, that black physicians tend to be more liberal than white physicians in their thinking about NHI (Colombotos, Kirchner, and Millman, 1975b; see also Richard, 1969).

7. These efforts lead to charges of "reverse discrimination," best exemplified by the famed Bakke case. In that case, the Supreme Court decided (1977) that the University of California acted unconstitutionally in reserving a set number of medical school admissions for non-whites whose academic qualifications might be lower than those of whites.

8. The 1940 U.S. data include foreign-born individuals. To check whether this distorts the comparison, we examined 1970 data that permit separate regional classification of native-born and foreign-born individuals; the two groups differed by no more than 1 percent. Another potential problem is the use of a single point of comparison (1940) to cover the wide age range of physicians, since the regions were growing at various rates during the relevant period. For example, the West increased 40 percent between 1940 and 1950, compared to a 10 percent increase in the Northeast. However, an elaborate analysis to compare separate cohorts is not justified for present purposes.

9. Recent research on women physicians has focused on their choice of specialties (i.e., sex-typing within an occupation), specifically in relation to traditional family roles and other sex-role expectations, their productivity, and other aspects of their career and life patterns (Ducker, 1974; Heins, 1979; Grenell, 1980; Lorber, 1981). Other studies have speculated about the impact of the growing number of women physicians on the profession and on health care (Shapiro and Jones, 1979).

10. The group of "other" religious backgrounds, as we have seen, is almost entirely made up of foreign physicians from the Far East.

11. Recall that the set of categories we use is white, black, oriental, and other. We should also point out that the base numbers in the nonwhite categories are small. There are 55 black respondents, 65 who are oriental, and 45 "other."

12. A note of caution: some part of these age differences may indicate individual career changes. For example, some young physicians may start out in salaried and group practice and then switch over to solo, fee-for-service practice. The pattern of age differences in board certification reflects both processes—individual career changes and long-term trends: the proportion who are board-certified was 27 percent among those under 35 years of age, 56 percent among those 35–64, and 28 percent among those 65 or over.

13. The figure reported for Puerto Rican students enrolled in medical schools in 1982–83 included those enrolled in the Commonwealth. We have excluded these students to make the statistics consistent with those of earlier years. It is of interest to note that in the late 1970s "other Hispanic" and "Asian or Pacific Islander" were added to the definition of "minority." The latter group has increased appreciably in recent years.

4 Social Background, Professional Characteristics, and Attitudes

We begin with an analytic framework for hypothesizing and explaining relationships between the social or professional characteristics of physicians and their attitudes. We view thse characteristics—for example, being working class in origin, Jewish, male, first-generation, mid-western, urban, in private practice, in pediatrics—as *social statuses* (defined as positions in a social system [Merton, 1957: 368]), and as sources of *socialization*. But we also consider that other mechanisms, such as social selection and self-interest, may account for differences in physicians' attitudes.

Mechanisms Linking Social Background, Professional Characteristics, and Attitudes

Socialization

We use the term "socialization" to designate "the processes by which people selectively acquire the *values* and *attitudes*, the interests, skills, and knowledge—in short, the culture—current in the *groups* of which they are, or seek to become, a member" (Merton, 1957: 287 [*emphasis added*]). The processes are grounded in socially patterned *experiences*.[1]

Socialization theory and research have focused on different *stages* of the life cycle—on childhood (McCandless, 1969), adolescence (Adelson, 1980), middle age (Levinson, 1978), and old age (Rosow, 1974); on different *content* areas—from political views and behavior (Renshon, 1977), to illicit drug use (Kandel, 1980), to professional values and performance (Merton, Reader, and Kendall, 1957); on different *agents* of socialization and social *settings*—the family (Gecas, 1981: 170–178), professional schools and other formal socializing organizations (Brim and Wheeler, 1966: 53–116; Mortimer and Simmons, 1978: 435–440) and occupations (Moore, 1969; Mortimer and Simmons, 1978: 440–443; Gecas, 1981: 187–191; Kohn and Schooler, 1983).

Early studies of socialization, mainly by psychologists, emphasized the effects of an individual's childhood experiences on later personality. Research since the 1960s, however, much of it conducted by sociologists, has studied socialization as it continues throughout the life cycle (see Becker, 1964; Rosow, 1965; and Brim and Wheeler, 1966; see also Sewell, 1963; Mortimer and Simmons, 1978; Bush and Simmons, 1981; Gecas, 1981).

Much of the socialization research on occupational and professional groups has focused on their *formal* training and education, possibly because students are more accessible to researchers than practicing professionals.[2] The term "professional socialization" is generally used to refer to this stage. A common theme of this research is the strong impact of professional school on the attitudes and behavior of students. Eron comments on "not only the profound changes taking place in students as they progress through four years of medical school, but *how alike they all appear at the end of those years*" [*emphasis added*] (1958: 25).

But, we argue, both earlier experiences and later work-related experiences may play important roles in shaping the characteristics and attitudes of individuals in addition to their experiences during formal training and education.

The significance of earlier sources of socialization in research on the professions is recognized in studies describing the social origins of business leaders, journalists, civil servants, public relations men, military leaders, teachers, physicians, nurses, and other professional groups. As we discussed in Chapter 3, these descriptions are included for a variety of reasons: to suggest why members of one profession may differ from those of another in a broad range of attitudes and behavior; to indicate the greater social status of one profession over another and its greater access to political power.[3] Few studies, however, examine the effects of specific social background characteristics on specific attitudes, behavior, and careers *within* a professional group.[4]

Similarly, the "socializing" effects of work and occupations have been the focus of much thinking and investigation, extending from the writings of Marx on the factory and alienation (see Bottomore and Rubel, 1956: 167–177), to empirical studies by Kohn and Schooler (1983) on the effects of job characteristics on psychological functioning. The fact of *intra-professional differentiation*, including its sources and its consequences, has been persuasively depicted by Bucher and Strauss (1961) and Freidson (1970: 87–108). But relatively little empirical research has been done on the effects of differentiated segments and worksettings within professional groups on the attitudes and behavior of their incumbents.[5]

Our focus in this chapter is the impact of these two relatively neglected sources of socialization—*early*, social background characteristics and *later*, professional characteristics—on the attitudes of physicians toward political and health care issues.

Freidson argues persuasively that the *present* "worksetting" of physicians has greater impact on their professional performance than their *prior* "socialization" (1970: 89–90):

> Far too much attention has been paid to the *personal characteristics* and attitudes of individual members of occupations and far too little to the *worksettings*.
>
> There is some very persuasive evidence that *"socialization"* does not explain some important elements of professional performance half so well as does the organization of the immediate work environment . . .
>
> Critical elements of professional behavior—the level of technical performance, the approach to the client, "cynicism" and ethicality—do not vary so much with the individual's *professional* training as with the social setting in which he works after his education. (*Emphasis added*)

Note that Freidson restricts the term "socialization" to designate experiences temporally *prior* to the "immediate work environment," as though the immediate work environment has no "socializing" effects on participants and as though these effects do not spill over and influence attitudes and behavior in other concurrent or subsequent social situations.[6] He thus minimizes the effects on individuals' attitudes and behavior of experiences in *prior* or other *concurrent* "immediate" social environments. People are portrayed almost as social chameleons, responding only to the direct and immediate pressures of one environment after another.[7]

The question could be posed as: What are the relative effects of "person" versus "environment," or of "prior socialization" versus "current worksetting," on attitudes and behavior? But we believe it is more fruitful to reformulate it to ask: What are the relative effects—*over time*—on attitudes and behavior of different social situations and experiences? We conceive of social situations and experiences as sources of *continuous* socialization. True, the effects of some of these experiences may recede over time, but the effects of others may persist. People have new experiences (e.g., medical school). The effects of some of these experiences "take" and supplant or moderate the effects of earlier experiences; the effects of others are deflected by the continuing impact of earlier experiences. Furthermore, the patterns of effects may vary depending on the *content* of attitudes and behavior. Freidson discusses professional performance and behavior; we examine attitudes toward a wide range of political and health care issues. (Many of the points just discussed are systematically examined by Bloom [1979: 36–46], in somewhat different terms, in an excellent review essay on theory and research on socialization for the physician's role.)

We use the socialization framework in several ways to provide a rationale for our hypotheses and explanations linking physicians' objective characteristics and their attitudes. First we examine attitudes that are distinctive of different statuses and consider how they impinge, directly or indirectly, on attitudes toward political and health care issues.

In some instances previous research has shown that attitudes vary among social groups *in the population*. Take, for example, the familiar finding that in the general population Jews are more likely than Protestants to be liberal politically. It could be argued that Jewish *physicians* are also more likely than Protestant *physicians* to be liberal. Or it could be argued that the influence of these social origins is obliterated by socialization into the profession. Underlying both arguments is the assumption that Jewish and Protestant physicians are representative of Jews and Protestants in the population with respect to political ideology—or, if they are not, that the direction and extent of the nonrepresentativeness are about the same in the two groups. For example, although Jewish physicians may be more conservative than other Jews, and Protestant physicians may be more conservative than other Protestants, the *relationship* between religious affiliation and political ideology is assumed to be about the same among those entering the medical profession as in the general population.[8]

The example of religious background illustrates the direct influence of membership in a group on attitudes toward the political and health care issues under investigation. The indirect impact of social background on an attitude under investigation requires the tracing of that influence *through* another attitude. Here we refer to a structure of related attitudes.

It has been shown, for example, that middle-class people are more likely than working-class people to value autonomy and independence (Gecas, 1979). If we assume that among *physicians*, an emphasis on autonomy and independence is associated with negative attitudes toward such issues as group practice and peer reviews, then we would expect physicians from middle-class backgrounds to be more likely than those from working-class backgrounds to oppose group practice and peer reviews.

Merton's analysis of the social dynamics of adaptation in "status-sets" and "status-sequences" puts the problem in more general terms (1957: 380–384):

> Primary socialization in certain statuses, with their characteristic value-orientations, may so affect the formation of personality as to make it sometimes more, sometimes less, difficult to act out the requirements of other statuses. (p. 381)

In the extreme case, socialization in a status inhibits (or ensures) the occupation of another status. For example, Christian Scientists hardly ever become physicians (Merton, 1957: 383). Or, a less extreme case, Catholics are underrepresented in psychiatry, and within psychiatry, in psychoanalysis (Lally, 1975).[9]

In the examples given so far, our rationale for expecting that a given objective characteristic is related to a given attitude is straightforward. The link in other examples, however, is more problematic. Why, for example, should we expect the religious background of physicians to be related to their attitudes toward peer reviews? And why should we expect their professional characteristics to be related to their political attitudes? What does it mean in terms of attitudes to be an academic physician rather than a clinical practitioner? To work in a salaried group practice rather than in a fee-for-service individual practice? To be a surgeon rather than a pediatrician? How do these experiences—the "conditions of work," the "demands of the job"—affect the attitudes of physicians toward political and health care issues? We shall discuss some of these rationales later in this chapter.

We are further confronted with the possibility that positions *within* a profession do not draw randomly from the entire pool of recruits into that profession. There may be *self*-selection and *institutional* selection, both in terms of the social characteristics of recruits (e.g., see Lally [1975] on the underrepresentation of Catholics in psychiatry) and their attitudes at the time of entering these positions.

Before turning to selection and other mechanisms, however, let us review some ways in which objective characteristics may be classified, other than as professional or nonprofessional and according to life-cycle stage. Then, let us discuss how these dimensions might affect the attitudes of physicians.

Types of Statuses

In Chapter 3 we distinguished between "professional" and "nonprofessional" characteristics. Professional characteristics are those that describe the physician's work situation; some of these (e.g., medical specialty) are unique to physicians, while others characterize the work of some non-physicians as well (e.g., working alone as an individual practitioner or in a group with colleagues).

Social, or demographic, characteristics (e.g., socioeconomic background) apply to the general population. The use of these variables in population studies is highly routinized, with good reason. They identify major divisions in the social structure, and they are associated with individuals' attitudes and behaviors toward a wide spectrum of issues (see Berelson and Steiner, 1964: 476–491; Bendix and Lipset, 1966: 353–499).

Although the distinction between social and professional characteristics and their temporal location in the life cycle are conceptually distinct, they are empirically linked. Professional statuses, even those that involve professional training, cannot be occupied until well into early adulthood, whereas social statuses can be occupied at birth. (Note the correspondence of this distinction with that between *achieved* and *ascribed* statuses.)

Social characteristics, however, may be *stable* extending throughout the individual's life cycle, or may *change*. Gender and ethnicity, for example, do not change—although the content and intensity of the influence of these statuses on their occupants' attitudes may change historically. Consider the growth of feminism. Examples of statuses that may change are discrepancies between socioeconomic origin and present socioeconomic status, or between national and regional origins and present place of practice. Physicians from working-class backgrounds and those raised in other countries or regions were exposed to influences that are presumably very different from those to which they are currently exposed.

They may resolve these differences by rejecting the influences of their past or their present; or by adopting attitudes "intermediate" between those characteristics of their "status of origin" and "status of destination"; or mobility may have a dynamic of its own—for example, persons who are mobile may "*over*conform."[10]

Professional statuses may also change. Physicians change specialties and worksettings. Again, changers may retain attitudes appropriate to their prior statuses, or they may conform to those characteristics of their new statuses. (They may even move from one status to another *because* they are dissatisfied with their old position, in part because they hold attitudes that are more appropriate to their new position than to the old one—a case of "selection.")

Another way in which statuses differ is whether they are a *continuous* source of socialization (e.g., socioeconomic status, gender, ethnicity) or whether they are *temporally circumscribed* (e.g., medical education, professional statuses) during an individual's lifetime. Although the *content* of "continuous" statuses may *change* (e.g., feminism), their impact continues uninterrupted from birth to death; temporally circumscribed statuses, however, have a beginning and/or an end *within* the life cycle.

On the other hand, the impact of a status is not limited to the period during which it is occupied—we have already implied that point in arguing the potential impact of earlier, though currently inactive, sources of socialization on current attitudes. Conversely, the impact of a status may *precede* the individual's occupation of that status, as captured in the concept "anticipatory socialization" (Merton, 1957: 265–268).

Types of Attitudes

Analogous to our distinction between professional and nonprofessional *statuses*, we distinguish between "professionally" and "nonprofessionally" relevant *attitudes*. The distinction corresponds somewhat to that between "health care" and "political issues," with "government-in-medicine" issues falling in between (see Chapter 2).

Political issues, such as general political ideology and attitudes toward general economic-welfare issues, are no more salient, we would argue, to physicians than they are to members of the general public. On the other hand, health care issues—group practice, physician reimbursement, method of payment, peer reviews, and task delegation—though of apparently increasing concern to the general public, are likely to be more salient to physicians because these issues impact on the organization of their daily work.[11]

What is the impact of different types of statuses on different types of attitudes? On the basis of our analysis of the formal properties of social statuses as sources of socialization, what can we say about their potential impact on current attitudes?

Early sources of socialization might seem to have the edge over late ones and current sources because of their temporal *primacy*; their prior, "unobstructed" access to the individual have an impact that resists later influences. On the other hand, later and current sources of socialization may have the edge because of their immediacy and their greater relevance to current issues. Which source predominates at any moment may depend on the issue—the object of the attitude.

We hypothesize that early socialization, located, for example, in ethnic and socioeconomic settings, has a greater effect on general and diffuse ("nonprofessional") attitudes, such as political ideology and on values such as autonomy, than on professionally relevant, work-specific attitudes, such as attitudes toward the formal organization of medical practice and peer reviews. (This general point is made by both Sewell [1963:

178] and by Brim and Wheeler [1966: 31–32].) These work-specific attitudes could be influenced indirectly by early sources of socialization to
the degree that they are parts of attitude structures that include general
and diffuse attitudes. To refer to an earlier example, it might be hypothesized that physicians from middle-class backgrounds are less likely than
those from working-class backgrounds to accept peer reviews because of
the greater emphasis on independence training in childhood in middle-
class homes. These early influences on work-specific attitudes are likely
to be weaker than those on nonprofessional attitudes because they must
operate "through" intervening nonprofessional attitudes (in the example
given, "independence").[12]

Conversely, later and current socialization in professional statuses (e.g.,
worksetting and specialty) have a greater effect, we expect, on attitudes
toward professionally relevant issues than on attitudes toward general,
nonprofessional issues. Whether, for example, physicians are in a group
or in an individual practice would seem to be more relevant to their
attitudes toward peer reviews than to their general political ideology; and
whether they are in a group or individual practice would seem to have a
greater impact on their attitudes toward peer reviews than whether they
were raised in a middle-class or working-class home.

What are the effects of the other properties of statuses on attitudes? We
expect that the longer and more stable the source of socialization, the
greater its impact. Thus, personal characteristics such as gender and
ethnic-religious background, pressing on individuals throughout their
lifetime, should have, *ceteris paribus*, a greater effect than their worktype
and specialty. And the less change from one category of a status to
another, the greater will be the effect of that status. Contrast, for example,
the effects of geopolitical environment and specialty on someone who has
lived all his/her life in the same area and practiced in the same specialty
with those on someone who has lived in different geographic areas or has
changed specialties.

Social Selection

So far in our discussion of socialization, the causal direction of the
relationship between objective social statuses and attitudes has been clear:
individuals exposed to the experiences, norms, and expectations in a
certain status are likely to adopt attitudes characteristic of that status. In
introducing the notion of "status-sequences," or "careers," we recognized
that attitudes characteristic of a certain status may be due, in part or in
whole, to the *prior* socialization of a disproportionate number of
members of that status in an earlier status. It is possible that psychiatrists,

for example, are more likely than general practitioners and other specialists to be politically liberal because they are more likely than other
specialists to be Jewish. To test this possibility we can control statistically
for the earlier status (e.g., religious background) and examine the relationship between a later status (e.g., specialty) and an attitude (e.g.,
political ideology).

This type of selection involves the *non*random recruitment of individuals into the medical profession or into its segments in terms of their prior,
objective personal (and usually stable) characteristics (discussed in Chapter 3). Another type of selection is in terms of the prior *attitudes* of
recruits. To continue with the previous example, it is possible that psychiatry *attracts* the more politically liberal medical students and housestaff,
regardless of their religious background. Thus, if a cross-sectional study
were to find interspecialty differences in political attitudes, we would not be
certain that these differences preceded (social selection) or followed (specialty-specific socialization experiences) entry into the specialties, because
we could not control for prior, potentially volatile attitudes. Short of a
longitudinal design, however, we shall turn later in this chapter to strategies for analyzing cross-sectional data to support one or the other interpretation. (For an excellent discussion of these strategies, see Hyman [1955:
198–226].)

A third type of nonrandom recruitment into the medical profession
focuses on selection in terms of prior attitudes "out of" a prior status rather
than "into" a status. We might label the former instance as selection out of
a status of "origin"; the latter, as selection into a status of "destination"
within the profession.

In our thinking about the relationship between social origins—such as
socioeconomic and religious-ethnic background and gender—and current
attitudes, there is no problem in establishing the time order between these
variables, as there is in examining the relationship between professional
statuses, such as specialty, and attitudes. Clearly the social origins come
first. There is no opportunity for physicians' self-selection *into* these statuses on the basis of prior attitudes.[13]

But we must consider the possibility that the medical profession attracts
from specific groups in the population people whose attitudes differ from
others in the group. Whereas the Jews it attracts, for example, may be more
conservative than those in the population, the non-Jews may be more
liberal than those in the population. In such a case we would find that
Jewish physicians are no more likely, or even less likely, than non-Jewish
physicians to be liberal.

Anticipating, then, the relationship between background characteristics
and present attitudes and behavior of a profession depends on the assumptions that are made not only about the degree to which specified attitudes

and behavior are distinctive of given groups in the population but also about the strength and direction of *differential* selection from those groups into the profession.

Self-Interest: A Complementary Formulation

Implicit in our discussion of the effects of the social and professional characteristics of physicians on their attitudes toward political and health care issues is their "self-interest." The disadvantaged, for example, are generally more sympathetic than the advantaged to changes in the social order because they think they have something to gain from these changes; the advantaged are more resistant because they have more to gain by maintaining the status quo than by changing it. Differences in attitudes are grounded, at least in part, in differences in the *interests* of persons occupying different social statuses.[14]

But the empirical relationship between peoples' social characteristics and their attitudes based on self-interest may persist long after changes in the conditions that generate these differences, both during the lifetimes of individuals and over succeeding generations. For example, apart from the historical propensity of Jews to identify with liberal causes (Cohn, 1958; Fuchs, 1958; Ladd and Lipset, 1975: 154–157), the Jewish Democratic vote in the 1930s was strengthened, it is argued, because of Roosevelt's stand against Hitler (Ladd and Hadley, 1978: 60–64); and the Democratic allegiance of urban, Catholic, ethnic groups is explained by the Democratic party's position on such issues as immigration and discrimination (Ladd and Hadley, 1978: 46–57). Continuing *intra*group ties (socialization) may sustain *inter*group differences in voting habits, attitudes toward specific issues, and ideology that are no longer based on such group interests.

Closely connected to this formulation is the idea of "ideology-by-proxy" suggested by Campbell and others (1960: 220). People cut their "information costs" by conforming to the political norms of groups of which they are members and with which they share self-interests that presumably generate these norms.

There are familiar occasions where self-interest operates in a more naked, direct, and short-term way, however, and dictates positions on specific issues that may run counter to people's ideology (see Campbell et al., 1960: 188–215). The response of physicians when asked what they thought about the idea that all physicians should get a regular salary—"What amount of salary did you have in mind?" (quoted in Chapter 2)—is an apt example. And, in our study of New York State practitioners, we found that the attitudes of physicians toward a full time county health department in areas without one was influenced by both their political ideology and, among part-time health officers, by their self-interest: liberals and those who would be least adversely affected by the establishment of a full-time county health department were more likely to support one than conservatives and those who would be most adversely affected (Colombotos, 1969b). Similarly, attitudes toward specific issues such as national health insurance, group practice, method of physician reimbursement, peer reviews, and the like may be influenced both by the socialization of physicians and by their professional norms and ideologies, on the one hand, and by immediate self-interests, on the other.

Guided by the foregoing general conceptual framework, we turn next to our hypotheses and findings linking the social background and professional practice characteristics of physicians to their attitudes.

Anticipated Relationships between Social Background, Professional Characteristics, and Attitudes

The Influence of Social Background Characteristics

The attitudes of Americans toward economic-welfare issues and, by extension, toward the role of government-in-medicine, differ according to their socioeconomic status, their ethnic-religious background, their generation-in-the-U.S., their gender, and the region of the country and the size of the city or town in which they live. With remarkable consistency over the past half-century, persons who are highly educated, affluent, Protestant, and white, those who, along with their parents (and grandparents), were born in the United States, men, and those living outside the Northeast and large cities are more likely to take conservative positions on these issues than persons who are less educated, less affluent, Catholics and Jews, black and other minority groups, recent immigrants, women, and those living in the Northeast and in large cities.[15]

The *specific* economic-welfare issues on which these groups differ range over a wide subject matter and their emphasis has changed over the decades with shifts in the focus of debate. In the 1940s, the issues focused on questions about labor unions, big business, and graduated income taxes; in the 1980s on questions about cuts in spending on food stamps, loans to college students, and national health insurance.

Moreover, it is argued that some of these group differences have been lessening in recent decades. The case is made that differences in political-economic attitudes according to socioeconomic status have been declining steadily since the mid-1940s and that they are likely to continue to decline (Campbell et al., 1960: 356–361; Abramson, 1975). An opposing view—that social class differences in political behavior have not declined since the 1930s—is argued by Alford (1963: 219–249). And, although it is commonly believed that regional and urban-rural differences in a wide variety of values and beliefs, including political attitudes, are becoming blurred, there is evidence of their persistence (Glenn and Simmons, 1967; Glenn and Hill, 1977).

We will not dwell on these refinements and qualifications, however. Our purpose is to see whether the *patterns* of relationships between social background characteristics and attitudes toward *political* and *government-in-medicine* issues that have been found in the general population also appear among physicians.

Studies of the public's attitudes toward *health care* issues, notably group practice, prepayment, and the use of nurse-practitioners and physicians' assistants, however, rarely report findings broken down by social background characteristics.

Moreover, the influence of social background characteristics on attitudes toward these health care issues may or may not be the same among the medical profession as it is among the general public. For example, both Jews in the medical profession and in the general population may regard peer review more favorably than their non-Jewish counterparts because they are more likely to have liberal political views; or, to take another example, support for group practice in the North Central states may be higher than in the other regions among both physicians and the public.

On the other hand, it could be argued that social background characteristics may impact on health care attitudes in quite different ways among physicians and the public. Physicians from lower-class backgrounds, for example, may be more likely than those from upper-class backgrounds to support group practice because of their lesser emphasis on individualism and autonomy, whereas these class-linked values may be less likely to affect the general public's attitudes.

In any case, we would argue that the overall influence of the social background characteristics of physicians on their health care attitudes is likely to be weaker than is the influence of their professional characteristics on those same attitudes.

The Influence of Professional Characteristics

In Chapter 3 we described how physicians differed in the content and organization of their work. Here, we examine how—and why—these characteristics, mainly their worksetting, specialty, and income level, are related to physicians' attitudes.

The general issue is whether differences in the content and conditions of physicians' work are of minor significance in relation to the common occupational identity and interests shared by all physicians or whether such differences override the sense of identity and interests. These alternatives have been formulated as different theories about professional unity and differentiation. One theory is the functionalist, or consensus, view, implicit in an early paper by Goode (1957); the other is a conflict view by Bucher and Strauss (1961).

Intraprofessional differentiation is recognized by both theoretical orientations, but is viewed very differently. In the first, differentiation derives from a functional division of labor and system of stratification, within a common value-system and a basic "community of interest." By contrast, Bucher and Strauss see differentiation as a continually shifting outcome of "diversity and conflict of interest" (1961: 325). They use the term "segments" to refer to such interest groups within professions, and illustrate with the differences among activity groups in medicine: "If, for example, the model physician is taken as one who sees patients and carries out the diagnosis and treatment of illness, then an amazing variety of physicians do not fit this model" (1961: 327).

In short, the perspectives of the "profession as community" and of the "professions in process" both recognize that objective differentiation, both vertical and horizontal, exists among individuals who are members of what is generally recognized as a single occupation. The "process" theorists place primary emphasis on work-differences in spite of a common occupational title and a set of nominally inclusive institutions; theorists of the profession as a "community" place greater emphasis on shared identity in spite of diversity in activities. To the extent that the difference between these theoretical orientations is merely one of relative emphasis, they can be seen as complementary, their relevance depending on the problem posed.

The containment of specialized and potentially conflicting interests remains a continuing problem for professional groups.[16] We shall return to this question in the final chapter. Here we are concerned with whether these segments differ in their political and health care views.

Worksetting

Our rationale for expecting *certain* professional characteristics to be related to *certain* attitudes is straightforward. For example, we expect physicians who actually are in group practice to be more likely to support that type of practice organization than those in individual practice. By extension, we expect the former to be more likely than the latter to accept "correlates," that is, features related to working in groups, such as peer reviews, delegation of tasks to nonmedical personnel, salaried reimbursement, and prepayment. Similarly, physicians in *salaried* group practice should be more likely than those in *fee-for-service* group practice to accept salaried practice. However, *salaried* group practitioners should be more likely than *fee-for-service* group practitioners to favor peer reviews, task delegation, and prepayment because they tend to be in larger groups compared with fee-for-service physicians and because large groups are more likely than small groups to have these features (see Wolinsky, 1982).

The rationale for these expectations is self-evident: the expected attitudinal differences correspond to, or parallel, objective differences in the worksettings of physicians. What remains problematic is the reason for that association. Is it self-selection or socialization? Are physicians with certain attitudes (e.g., pro-group practice) attracted to, selected by, and retained in, certain settings, or do experiences in certain settings generate and sustain attitudes compatible with working in these settings?

Further, we expect physicians working outside of patient care activities—teachers, administrators, researchers—to take relatively liberal positions on the health care issues we investigated. But the rationale is, again, problematic. Most of these issues deal with patient care, an activity to which these physicians do not commit the major portion of their time. Thus, it could be argued that nonpractitioners are relatively liberal on these issues because they are not directly affected—they have "nothing to lose." Or, it could be argued that they are relatively liberal because almost without exception the situations they work in (i.e., salaried positions in organizations) contain the same elements represented in the health care issues—salaried employment, peer reviews, and a complex division of labor.

Still another view sees nonpractitioners differing from practitioners in their attitudes toward health care issues because of differences in their ideology. In a qualitative field study of relationships between medical faculty and medical practitioners in eight communities, it was noted that medical faculty (teachers and some researchers in our worksetting categories) were considerably more receptive to change in a variety of professional spheres, including new ways of organizing medical practice (Kendall, 1965: 228–232). Public health physicians are also presumed to be more liberal in their thinking than practitioners (Rosen, 1961; Back, 1968).[17]

Turning to attitudes toward political and government-in-medicine issues, we expect physicians in nonpatient care activities and those in salaried, group practice to be the most likely to take liberal positions, followed by physicians in fee-for-service group pratice and physicians in fee-for-service individual or partnership practice, in that order. Our rationale is that physicians in "nontraditional" practice settings and activities are more likely than those in "traditional" settings and activities to take "nontraditional" positions, in general, on a wide range of political and health care issues.

Implicit in this rationale is the larger question of whether people differ in their general orientation toward change and innovation in a way that spills over to influence their attitudes toward a wide range of specific issues (Campbell et al., 1960: 209–212).

Finally, physicians in different worksettings differ in a number of other ways, such as professional prestige and income, that may explain their attitudes toward political and health care issues. Salaried group practitioners earn less than fee-for-service practitioners. Health officers have less prestige and earn less income than practitioners. Academic physicians have more prestige, but earn less, than practitioners.

Specialty

Physicians in different specialties differ in their personalities and in their personal values. (For a review of this literature, based mainly on specialty choices of medical students, see Otis et al., 1974; Zuckerman, 1977; USD-HEW, 1978.) As viewed by medical students, surgeons are domineering and arrogant, aggressive and mainly concerned with their own prestige; internists are sensitive to a wide range of factors in evaluating medical problems and deeply interested in intellectual problems; general practitioners are deeply interested in people, patient, and friendly; psychiatrists are also deeply interested in intellectual problems and they are emotionally unstable and confused in their thinking (Bruhn and Parsons, 1964).

More relevant to our purpose here, specialties also differ with respect to other properties—professional status and income, the intensity of interaction between practitioners and patients, the organization of their work ("worksetting"), and the problems with which they deal.

SOCIAL PRESTIGE AND INCOME. Prestige ratings by physicians, medical and other university students, and patients generally place surgical specialties at the top of the prestige hierarchy and general practice and psychiatry near the bottom (Reader, 1958: 177; Schwartzbaum and McGrath, 1972; Shortell, 1974). Following surgical specialties are, roughly in this order: internists, pediatricians, radiologists-pathologists-anesthesiologists, and specialties generally grouped in an "all other" category—such as those in aerospace medicine, occupational medicine, physical medicine and rehabilitation, preventive medicine, and public health.[18] Closely corresponding to these prestige ratings is physicians' income; surgeons earn the highest incomes while general practitioners and psychiatrists are among those who earn the lowest incomes.

We expect that the high-prestige and high-income specialists, because they are more satisfied with their careers and generally content with the status quo, will be more likely than the low-prestige and low-income specialists to hold conservative views on political and health care issues.[19]

SOCIAL INTERACTION BETWEEN PHYSICIAN AND PATIENT. Specialties differ in the degree of social interaction between physician and patient and in the potential for patient influence in the encounter. General practitioners, internists, pediatricians, and psychiatrists interact more intensively with their patients than do surgeons, anesthesiologists, radiologists, and pathologists.[20]

We expect that the higher the level of interaction between patients and practitioners, the greater is the likelihood that physicians see their patients as "persons" rather than as circumscribed "disease entities" and that physicians in high-interaction specialties are in turn more likely than those in low-interaction specialties to be socialized by their patients. Since the general population is more likely than the medical profession to hold politically liberal views, it would follow that high-interaction specialists are more likely than low-interaction specialists to adopt the relatively liberal political views of their patients.[21]

SPECIALTIES AND THE ORGANIZATION OF THEIR WORK. Specialties vary greatly in the organization of their work (worksetting). General practitioners are overrepresented in the solo and partnership, fee-for-service category. Anesthesiologists, radiologists, and obstetricians-gynecologists are overrepresented in fee-for-service groups and pathologists and psychiatrists in salaried group practice.

We expect that, *controlling for their own worksetting,* physicians in specialties characterized by more organized settings are more likely than those in specialties characterized by more traditional settings to have liberal views, primarily in their health care attitudes and secondarily in their political and government-in-medicine attitudes.

The proportion of physicians in each specialty who are in each worksetting is viewed as a part of the *social context* of that specialty and presumed to influence the attitudes of those specialists above and beyond the influence of their own individual worksettings.[22]

SPECIALTY-SPECIFIC VALUES. Specialties differ in the medical problems they deal with and develop distinctive sets of values to deal with these problems. Bucher and Strauss (1961) view professional segments (which include specialties and subgroups within them) as taking on the character of "social movements." They carve out distinctive missions, emphasize distinctive "ideologies," activities, methods, and techniques over others, form colleague networks, and recruit and socialize neophytes to their distinctive "schools" of thought.

Distinctive value systems that characterize different specialties may be more compatible with certain political and health care attitudes than with others.[23] It could be argued, for example, that physicians who view diseases as having primarily a social or environmental etiology are more likely than those who view them as having primarily a genetic, or hereditary, etiology to take liberal positions on political issues. (See Pastore [1948], who found such an association between scientists' views on the environmental-heredity issue and on social and political issues.)

On these grounds, psychiatrists, pediatricians, and physicians in public health, preventive medicine, and occupational medicine are expected to have more liberal views than other specialists.

CONTENT-SPECIFIC INTERESTS. Finally, specialists may respond differently to concrete programs. We expected, for example, general practitioners to be more likely than specialists to oppose Medicare and national health insurance. In England, the opposition of general practitioners to the National Health Service was rooted in the fear that the gap between them and the specialists in terms of status and income would be widened with the advent of the NHS and with subsequent changes in the program (see Eckstein, 1960).

Specialties vary with respect to each of the properties we have discussed; and different properties of a given specialty may push the members of that specialty in different directions with respect to their political and health care views. On the grounds that general practitioners have low status and low income and that their work involves a high level of interaction with patients, we would expect them to have liberal views; on the grounds, however, that they are concentrated in solo or partnership fee-for-service, we would expect them to have conservative views. Although obstetricians have moderately high status, which would make them conservative, their practice involves a high level of interaction with their patients, which would make them liberal. Although anesthesiologists, radiologists, and pathologists are overrepresented in organized settings, which would make them liberal, their work involves minimal interaction with patients, which would make them conservative.

Looking ahead to our analysis, we reduced the 22 specialty categories obtained in our interviews into five major, conventionally used categories: general/family practice, surgical, medical, psychiatry, and all other. These five categories are then used in both the contingency table analysis and in the multiple regression.

Next we ranked each of the 22 specialties according to its prestige level, average income level, average level of interaction between practitioner and patient, and a score based on the distribution of worksettings in that specialty. (We did not attempt to rate the specialties according to their "values" or "interests.") In the multiple regression, each physician was then assigned these four scores depending on his/her specialty. This method permits us to see how each of these four properties of physicians' specialties influences their political and health care views.

Income

We expect that, as with prestige, the higher the physicians' income the more likely they are to take conservative positions on political and health care issues, on the assumption that they have more at stake in maintaining the status quo.

Findings

We present our data in two ways. The first is a set of two-way contingency tables between each social background and professional characteristic and each attitude (Tables 4-1 and 4-2). The second is a hierarchical multiple regression analysis (Table 4-3).

Cross-Tabulation Analysis

In summary, Tables 4-1 and 4-2 show the following: The social background characteristics of physicians had a stronger impact on their attitudes toward political and government-in-medicine issues than on their attitudes toward health care issues; the latter were barely affected by social background. Especially notable is the influence of the religious background of physicians and their generational status in the United States. Equally notable is the absence of any influence of physicians' socioeconomic background.

Physicians' professional characteristics, on the other hand, influence their attitudes toward political and government-in-medicine issues about as much as do their social background characteristics, and about as much as they influence their attitudes toward health care issues. The workset-

Table 4-1. Physicians' Attitudes Toward Political and Health Care Issues by Their Social Background Characteristics[a]

		Political ideology (% liberal)	Gov't. in medicine (% liberal)	Group practice (% favor)	Peer reviews (% favor)	Task delegation (% favor)	Physician reimbursement: Salaried/ capitation (% accept)	Prepayment (% accept)
	Base N's							
Socioeconomic background								
Low (3–6) (1)	338	38	41	32	36	36	29	42
(7–10) (2)	832	42	45	35	40	39	30	42
(11–14) (3)	757	37	46	41	44	45	31	45
High (15–17) (4)	274	47	52	46	42	44	37	41
Father was MD (5)	385	36	43	36	35	44	25	41
$r =$		—	—	-.05	—	-.07	—	—
Religious background								
Protestant	1380	28	36	35	38	44	27	41
Catholic	623	39	50	39	37	37	30	40
Jewish	490	71	64	37	43	37	35	46
None, other	209	51	52	54	46	45	40	48
Eta $=$		.36	.24	.09	—	.09	.11	.07
Generation in U.S.								
First (1)	352	60	66	55	35	34	42	46
Second (2)	687	51	50	33	40	36	32	42
Third-or-more (3)	1650	32	40	36	41	45	27	42
$r =$		.22	.20	.08	—	-.10	.11	.05
Gender								
Male (2)	2573	39	45	37	40	41	30	42

		N							
Female	(1)	140	60	51	50	30	34	40	37
	r =		.11	—	—	.06	—	.05	—
Region									
North Central		621	36	39	39	37	38	28	39
South		767	37	39	35	36	43	25	36
West		564	37	42	37	43	46	26	47
East		761	48	60	40	42	37	39	48
	Eta =		.13	.19	—	—	—	.16	.15
Degree of urbanization									
Low (up to 50,000)	(1)	476	29	32	34	30	42	27	39
Medium (SMSA to 1 million)	(2)	949	32	41	36	41	44	25	40
High (SMSA 1 million or over)	(3)	1288	49	54	40	42	38	35	46
	r =		-.18	-.19	-.10	-.09	—	-.07	-.10
Age									
Under 35	(1)	306	51	54	50	55	55	34	49
35–44	(2)	847	42	47	42	46	46	29	42
45–54	(3)	785	37	42	34	37	41	30	40
55–64	(4)	527	34	43	34	33	32	27	41
65-or-over	(5)	248	40	48	25	20	27	33	44
	r =		.07	.07	.17	.20	.20	—	.04

aSee "Measures and Scales" in the Appendix for a description of the variables used in these tables.

In Tables 4-1, 4-2, and 5-1, we use "Eta," produced by analysis of variance, when the independent variables are nominal (religion, region, and specialty) and Pearson's r when they are ordinal (all the other independent variables). Eta^2 is directly analogous to r^2 in that they both indicate the proportion of variation in the dependent variable explained by the independent variable. The Eta's and r's are based on the raw attitude scores for each category of the independent variable. Rather than display the mean scores in Tables 4-1, 4-2, and 5-1, however, we show the proportion of physicians in each category who took a "liberal" position on each issue. Liberal positions, those characterizing the most liberal 30 to 40 percent of the total physician sample, are assigned low scores in calculating r and Eta.

Only r's and Eta's significant at the .01 level are shown in Tables 4-1, 4-2, and 5-1.

Table 4–2. Physicians' Attitudes Toward Political and Health Care Issues by Their Professional Characteristics[a]

Worksetting		Base N's	Political ideology (% liberal)	Gov't. in medicine (% liberal)	Group practice (% favor)	Peer reviews (% favor)	Task delegation (% favor)	Physician reimbursement: Salaried capitation (% accept)	Prepayment (% accept)
Patient Care									
Individual, fee-for-service	(1)	986	34	37	13	28	31	23	32
Group, or hosp.-based, fee-for-service	(2)	796	33	41	38	40	39	20	38
Group, or hosp.-based, salaried	(3)	465	50	56	60	48	52	45	51
Nonpatient care (teaching, research, administration)	(4)	415	58	65	66	57	57	50	64
	r =		-.20	-.24	-.47	-.26	-.23	-.24	-.27

		N	1	2	3	4	5	6	7
Specialty									
General/family practice		566	33	34	23	21	34	25	33
Surgical specialties		851	31	39	30	38	39	21	36
Medical specialties		585	49	54	46	49	45	35	44
Psychiatry		222	64	69	40	46	44	49	56
All other specialties		461	42	51	58	51	46	36	55
	Eta =		.25	.24	.29	.28	.14	.29	.22
Board certification									
Board-certified	(2)	1298	38	48	40	47	44	28	45
Not board-certified	(1)	1415	41	44	35	32	38	32	40
	r =		—	-.06	-.09	-.16	-.09	.04	-.07
Income									
Low (up to $30,000)	(1)	819	51	53	44	40	47	41	49
Medium ($30–49,999)	(2)	1054	37	45	35	41	42	29	43
High ($50,000 or more)	(3)	762	34	39	24	38	35	21	36
	r =		.14	.11	.19	—	.08	.18	.13

[a]See notes to Table 4-1.

ting and specialty of physicians are especially notable for their impact across the range of attitudes examined.

The direction of the relationships between the objective characteristics of physicians and their attitudes were essentially as expected. Among social background characteristics: Jewish physicians were by far the most liberal politically, followed by Catholics and then Protestants; first-generation physicians were more liberal than second- and third-generation physicians; women were slightly more liberal than men; and easterners and urbanites were more liberal than noneasterners and those who lived in rural areas.[24]

It is interesting to note that differences in the "distance" between the three generation categories varied according to the attitudes examined (see Table 4-1). On health care issues, second- and third-or-more-generation physicians, nearly all of whom were trained in the United States, were quite similar but differed from first-generation physicians, nearly all of whom were trained abroad. On political and government-in-medicine issues, however, differences among the three generation categories were more evenly spaced.

Younger physicians were considerably more liberal than their older colleagues in their thinking about the "organizational" issues of group practice, peer reviews, and task delegation, but they did not differ from their older colleagues in their attitudes toward the "economic" issues of salaried reimbursement and prepayment. And, younger physicians were barely more liberal than older physicians in their attitudes toward political and government-in-medicine issues. (The age of physicians is entered in the multiple regression as a control. We focus on the relationship between the age of physicians and their attitudes more closely in Chapter 5, which examines generational differences.)

Among professional characteristics, the influence of worksetting was precisely what we expected. Physicians in activities other than patient care (research, teaching, administration) were the most liberal in their attitudes toward all issues, and those in individual, fee-for-service practice were the most conservative. (Since researchers, teachers, and administrators differed little among themselves, they were combined into a single category in Table 4-2 and in the multiple regression.) In between, physicians in *salaried* group practice were more liberal than those in *fee-for-service* group practice.*

With respect to specialty, psychiatrists were the most liberal politically and general practitioners and surgeons were closely tied for being the

---

* The attitudes of the special sample of medical faculty in 11 schools and of the two special samples in prepaid group practice (see "Sampling Designs" in the Appendix) were similar to those in nonpatient care and salaried group practice, respectively, in Table 4-2.

most conservative. Those in the medical specialties and in the "all other" category were in-between. With respect to the health care issues the pattern is a bit erratic: general practitioners emerged as the most conservative, followed by surgeons, but psychiatrists and physicians in the "all other" category shared being the most liberal across the five issues.

Finally, the higher the physicians' income, the more conservative. Also, board-certified physicians, who earned higher incomes than those not certified, tended to be more liberal than those not certified.

Results from other surveys of physicians are generally consistent with the findings in Tables 4-1 and 4-2.[25]

Hierarchical Multiple Regression Analysis

A hierarchical multiple regression analysis, the second step of our analysis, permits us to examine the relationship between two variables (e.g., religious background and political ideology) efficiently controlling for other associated independent variables and to assess the relative importance of the independent variables in relation to each attitude. Hierarchical regression also requires us to make more explicit our conceptualization of the process linking the social and professional characteristics of physicians and their attitudes (displayed in Figure 4-1). It also pulls together the threads of our earlier discussion in this chapter.[26]

We carry out a regression analysis on each of the seven issues discussed so far—political ideology, government-in-medicine, and the five health care issues—as a dependent variable. Recognizing that establishing the temporal priority of attitudes in a cross-sectional study is problematic at best, we nevertheless view the three sets of attitudes as having "causal" interrelations. We assumed that in the development of physicians' thinking, their political ideology "precedes" their attitudes on government-in-medicine issues, where politics and health care intersect, and that these, in turn, "precede" their attitudes toward relatively "nonpolitical" health care issues. This conceptualization is represented in Figure 4-1.

The Causal Model

We begin, at Step 1 (see Figure 4-1), with the social origins of physicians—their religious background and generation-in-the-United States, their socioeconomic background, and gender. Age is included in this analysis as a control variable.

We hypothesized that the social background characteristics of physicians influence their political and health care attitudes through their

Figure 4-1. Causal Model: Social and Professional Characteristics and Attitudes

1	2	3	4	5	6	7	8	9
							Current Attitudes	
Social Background Characteristics	Early Politics	Career Values, Political Party in Medical School	Present Social Charac-teristics	Professional Charac-teristics	Satis-faction			
Religious Background	Father's Political Identification	Money	Region	Worksetting	Sat. with Income	Political Ideology	Gov't in Medicine	Group Practice
Socioeconomic (SEB)		Autonomy	Urban-ization	Specialty	General Prof. Sat.			Peer Reviews
Generation in U.S.		Political Party in Medical School		Board Certification				Task Delegation
Gender				Income				Physician Reimbursement
Age								Prepayment

98

fathers' political views and their own early political views and career values. Hence, we introduce these variables in Steps 2 and 3 of the model. Physicians who are Jewish, first generation, from lower-class backgrounds, and women would be more likely than those with contrasting attributes to have liberal political views and, through these, liberal views on government-in-medicine issues, in part because their fathers were more likely to be liberal and because they themselves started out with more liberal views in medical school.

Some of these social characteristics, we reasoned, might also operate through career values and professional characteristics to influence attitudes toward health care issues. Men are more likely than women to emphasize autonomy ("freedom from supervision") and money and prestige in their decision to go into medicine; physicians from upper- and middle-class backgrounds are more likely than those from working-class backgrounds to emphasize autonomy and less likely to emphasize money and prestige (on the relationship between socioeconomic background and emphasis on money and prestige, see Colombotos, 1969c). These, in turn, would influence their choice of worksetting and health care attitudes: those stressing autonomy and money would be less likely to enter salaried positions and hence less likely to take liberal positions on the health care issues.

In Step 4 we introduce geographic location factors, that is, where physicians currently live and practice, in terms of the region of the country and level of urbanization. Although these variables and professional characteristics, in the next step, both refer to the present, we separated them because we wanted to be able to identify their unique effects.

The worksetting of physicians, specialty, income level, and whether they are board-certified are introduced in Step 5. These characteristics may influence the health care attitudes of physicians indirectly by operating through their political and government-in-health attitudes, or they may influence health care attitudes directly. In both instances, the satisfaction of physicians with their careers in general and with their income in particular may intervene between their professional characteristics and their attitudes: the more satisfied, the more conservative.[27] Hence, these two types of satisfaction are added in Step 6.

Table 4-3 shows the initial and final standardized regression coefficients (beta's) significant at the .01 level and the multiple correlation coefficients squared (R^2), which indicate the amount of variation explained by the independent variables up to that point in the regression analysis. The initial beta's indicate the effect of an independent variable on a dependent variable when the former is first introduced in the

Table 4-3. Standardized Regression Coefficients, and R^2's in Hierarchical Multiple Regression (n = 1,478)[a]

	Dependent Variables													
	1 Political Ideology		2 Gov't in Medicine		3 Group Practice		4 Peer Reviews		5 Task Delegation		6 Physician Reimbursement		7 Prepayment	
	When first entered	Last step	When first entered	Last step	When first entered	Last step	When first entered	Last step	When first entered	Last step	When first entered	Last step	When first entered	Last step
First step														
Socioeconomic background (low SEB = 3; high = 17)[b]														
Religious background														
Protestant														
Catholic										−.08			.18	
Jewish	−.24	−.11	−.16											
[None, other]														
Generation in U.S.	.08													
Gender (women = 1, men = 2)	.08													
Age	.08	.11		−.06	.18		.23	.17	.23	.17				
	$R^2 = .15$		$R^2 = .07$		$R^2 = .05$		$R^2 = .06$		$R^2 = .07$		$R^2 = .01$		$R^2 = .01$	

Second step							
Father's political identification	.24	.14	.12		.08		.08
	$R^2 = .20$	$R^2 = .08$	$R^2 = .08$	$R^2 = .05$	$R^2 = .07$	$R^2 = .01$	$R^2 = .02$
Third step							
Career values: reason for choosing medicine							
Money (very important = 1, not at all = 5)					−.08	−.10	−.09
Autonomy (very important = 1, not at all = 5)	−.08		−.09	−.16	−.15	−.09	−.10
Political party in medical school	.39	.38	.12	.11	.11		
	$R^2 = .34$	$R^2 = .10$	$R^2 = .08$	$R^2 = .10$	$R^2 = .08$	$R^2 = .05$	$R^2 = .06$
Fourth step							
Region							
North central	.10	.11	.11		.09	.17	.08
South		.13	.09		.12	.16	.12
West		.08	.12		.08		
[East]							
Urbanization (low urban = 1, high urban = 9)	−.11	−.11	−.08		−.07	−.07	
	$R^2 = .35$	$R^2 = .13$	$R^2 = .10$	$R^2 = .11$	$R^2 = .08$	$R^2 = .07$	$R^2 = .08$

Table 4-3. (Continued)

	Dependent Variables													
	1 Political Ideology		2 Gov't in Medicine		3 Group Practice		4 Peer Reviews		5 Task Delegation		6 Physician Reimbursement		7 Prepayment	
	When first entered	Last step	When first entered	Last step	When first entered	Last step	When first entered	Last step	When first entered	Last step	When first entered	Last step	When first entered	Last step
Fifth step													
Worksetting													
[Solo, ffs]													
Group, ffs.	−.07	−.07	−.13	−.11	−.29	−.28	−.13	−.10	−.16	−.13	−.17	−.13	−.15	−.11
Group, salaried	−.12	−.12	−.14	−.11	−.37	−.34	−.13	−.10	−.16	−.13	−.21	−.16	−.21	−.16
Nonpatient care			−.19	−.14	−.39	−.35	−.14	−.09						
Specialty													
[General/family practice]													
Surgical			−.10	−.09	−.12	−.10	−.12	−.12						
Medical	−.07	−.07	−.13	−.09			−.20	−.18						
Psychiatry							−.13	−.10					−.10	
All other			−.10	−.09	−.10	−.10	−.18	−.18						
Board-certified (no = 1, yes = 2)					−.07				−.08				−.07	
Income	.07	.07			.07								.08	
	$R^2 = .39$		$R^2 = .20$		$R^2 = .32$		$R^2 = .19$		$R^2 = .13$		$R^2 = .15$		$R^2 = .16$	

Sixth step
  Satisfaction with
    income (high sat.
    = 1, low = 5)
  General professional
    satisfaction
    (high sat. = 2,
    low = 10)

	$R^2 = .40$	$R^2 = .20$	$R^2 = .32$	$R^2 = .19$	$R^2 = .13$	$R^2 = .16$	$R^2 = .16$
	−.07	−.07					

Seventh step

Political ideology	.43 .43	.13	.19 .10	.17 .11	.24 .16	.22 .13
	$R^2 = .31$	$R^2 = .33$	$R^2 = .21$	$R^2 = .15$	$R^2 = .19$	$R^2 = .19$

Eight step

Gov't in medicine	.14 .14	.14 .14	.21 .21	.14 .14	.20 .20	.22 .22
	$R^2 = .34$	$R^2 = .24$	$R^2 = .16$	$R^2 = .22$	$R^2 = .23$	

aMissing values in the regression were resolved by listwise deletion: a respondent was deleted from the analysis if there was a "no answer" on *any* variable. This procedure reduced the number of cases from 2,715 to 1,478. The variable means for the total sample and the MR sample were remarkably similar, suggesting that there was no serious bias in the surviving MR sample.

[ ] indicates reference category in dummy variables.

Only beta's significant at the .01 level are shown in this table.

See "Measures and Scales" in the Appendix for a description of the variables used. "Liberal" positions are assigned low scores.

bThose with physician-fathers are not identified separately in this scale.

regression analysis, controlling for the other independent variables entered up to and included in that step; the final beta's indicate the effect of an independent variable controlling for all other independent variables in the analysis. We have already discussed how the social and professional characteristics of physicians are related (in Chapter 3) and how their attitudes are related (in Chapter 2).

Using the causal terminology of the model, we see (in Table 4-3) that the political ideology of physicians influenced their attitudes toward government-in-medicine issues quite strongly (beta $= .43$); its effects on their health care attitudes, operating in part through their government-in-medicine views, were considerably weaker. Physicians' attitudes toward government-in-medicine, in turn, had a much stronger effect than political ideology on their attitudes toward health care issues, as indicated by the final beta's. This pattern is consistent with our analysis of attitude structure based on intercorrelations and factor analysis, in Chapter 2.

Consistent with our findings in Tables 4-1 and 4-2, the social background characteristics of physicians (in Step 1) explained more of the variation in their political ideology than in their attitudes toward health care issues. (The R^2 is .15 for political issues, .07 for government-in-medicine, and ranges between .07 and .01 for health care issues.) Present social background characteristics (Step 4: Region and Urbanization) added little explanatory power. On the other hand, when the professional characteristics of physicians were entered (in Step 5), they added more to explaining the variation in their health care attitudes than in their political ideology. (The increases in R^2 range from .05 for task delegation to .22 for group practice; the increase in R^2 for political ideology is only .04.)

In general, the specific findings of the regression analysis are consistent with those in the cross-tabular analysis, except for a few relationships that dropped below the .01 significance level with the application of statistical controls. More important, however, the hierarchical regression analysis permits us to explain some of these relationships.

The influence of physicians' religious upbringing and of their generational status in the United States on their current political ideology operated through their father's political thinking and their own early political views. The pathways of this influence differ a bit for religious upbringing and U.S.-generational status, however. The religious upbringing of physicians influenced their early political thinking both directly and indirectly, through their father's political thinking; their generational status, however, influenced their early political thinking only indirectly, through their father's thinking.

In contrast to the sharp effects of religious upbringing and the moderate effects of generation-in-the-United States, the socioeconomic background of physicians was unrelated to their political views. These results are generally consistent with those obtained by Ladd and Lipset on the influence of religious-ethnic and socioeconomic background on the political views of academics (1975: 149–180). There, too, religious background had a strong influence, with Jewish academics being the most liberal. Socioeconomic origins had a weak influence; in fact, those from high socioeconomic backgrounds were slightly more likely to hold *liberal* views than those from low socioeconomic backgrounds. The latter relationship, however, was explained entirely by subsequent career lines: academics from high socioeconomic backgrounds were more likely to be at major colleges and universities, where the subculture was more liberal, and less likely to be in the conservative disciplines. When type of institution and field were held constant, academics did not differ in their political views according to their socioeconomic backgrounds.[28]

With respect to physicians' gender, the more liberal general political ideology of women is explained by an accumulation of intervening variables, mainly by their being more likely to be in salaried settings than in individual practice and by earning lower incomes. They are no more likely than men to have entered medical school with liberal views. Conversely, *after* controlling for these and other factors, it turns out that men were *more* liberal in their views toward government-in-medicine.

Rural physicians were more conservative than urban physicians in their attitudes toward government-in-medicine and certain health care issues (group practice, reviews, and prepayment), in part because they were more likely to be in individual, fee-for-service practice and in general practice. On the other hand, rural physicians were more likely to favor the delegation of tasks after controlling for these same variables. Perhaps this is explained by lesser competition among physicians in rural areas than among those in urban areas.

Finally, older physicians were more likely than younger physicians to hold conservative views toward political and selected health care issues (peer reviews, the delegation of tasks, and to a lesser extent, group practice), in part because they were in individual and general practice and because they earned higher incomes, but physicians' age continued to have a direct effect on their attitudes toward peer reviews and task delegation, once these and all other variables in our model were controlled.

Among professional characteristics, the worksetting of physicians had the strongest and most consistent effects on their attitudes. Physicians in activities other than patient care and salaried group practitioners were, in that order, the most liberal in their views; solo, fee-for-service practitioners were the most conservative. The differences are especially striking in relation to health care issues, with beta's reaching as high as .39. It is noteworthy that the worksetting of physicians influenced their health care attitudes directly, and only slightly through their political and government-in-health attitudes.[29]

The "distance" between the three practitioner groups (solo, fee-for-service; group, fee-for-service; and group, salaried) in their attitudes toward health care issues (as indicated by the unstandardized regression coefficients) depends on the particular issue presented. *Group, fee-for-service* practitioners were closer to *individual, fee-for-service* practitioners than to *group, salaried* practitioners in their attitudes toward the "economic" issues of salaried reimbursement and prepayment; but they were closer to group, salaried practitioners in their attitudes toward the "organizational" issues of group practice, peer reviews, and task delegation.

In contrast to the strong and clear effects of physicians' worksettings on their attitudes were the effects of their specialty. Although the general pattern of differences was in the same direction as that in the cross-tabular analysis, only a few reached statistical significance: psychiatrists were still the most politically liberal specialty and general practitioners still stand out as the most clearly resistant to peer reviews.

But we learn little from this analysis about why specialties differ in their attitudes. To pursue this objective, we entered in the regression model four analytic variables to characterize each of the 22 specialties obtained in the interview, each of which we have discussed earlier in this chapter: social prestige of specialty, average income of physicians in specialty, an index based on the proportion of physicians in specialty distributed among the four worksettings, and experts' ratings of the typical degree of interaction between patients and physicians in each specialty.

Of the 28 regression coefficients (four dimensions of specialties × seven attitudes), only four were significant at the .01 level. Why specialists differ in their attitudes remains an intriguing question.

With respect to the income of physicians, the higher it is, the more politically conservative, but not because high-income physicians were more satisfied than low-income physicians. Low income and general professional dissatisfaction each led to liberal political views.[30] Finally, as in the tabular analysis, board-certified physicians tended to be more liberal than those who were not board-certified with respect to government-in-medicine and selected health care issues.

Socialization Versus Selection

There remains, in a cross-sectional design such as the one on which these data are based, the nagging question of whether relationships among physicians' worksettings, specialty, and other current professional characteristics, on the one hand, and their attitudes, on the other, are due to the effects of experiences identified by those characteristics (socialization) or to prior differences in the attitudes of those who choose different types of careers in medicine (selection). We discussed these different mechanisms earlier in the chapter.

Data provided by two analytic strategies applied to our cross-section suggest that although there is slight evidence of selection into different worksettings and specialties, socialization in these statuses has a stronger effect on the attitudes of physicians than does their original selection of worksetting and specialty:

1. Among senior physicians, their worksetting and specialty were less strongly correlated with their past political party preference, when they "started medical school," than with their current political party preference and general political ideology.
2. The correlation coefficients and standardized regression coefficients between fourth-year medical students' *plans* for entering different worksettings and specialties, on the one hand, and their current political and health care attitudes, on the other, were generally weaker than those between *current* worksettings and specialties of physicians and their attitudes toward these same issues.[31]

Summary

We noted earlier in this chapter the surge of interest in the last decade or two in socialization through the life cycle, balancing previous emphasis on childhood experiences and their presumed lasting impact on attitudes and values. With particular reference to professionals, it is commonly argued that with lengthier and increasingly more intensive professional training, the effects of early background on individuals' attitudes, behavior, and careers are obliterated.

Others have taken the argument one step further. They point out even the effects of professional training fade in the face of the immediate pressures of the *current* social setting of work. Our findings do, indeed, substantiate the impact of the latter on current attitudes toward health care issues.

But our findings also indicate that with respect to some types of attitudes the effects of early (and, in some cases, continuing) nonprofessional sources of socialization cannot be summarily dismissed. Differences in the political views of sociodemographic groups entering the profession correspond, with some exceptions, to differences in the views of those groups in the general population, and moreover, these differences persist over time.

Physicians are not "homogenized"; they are not all socialized to think alike. Clearly, Eron's observation about "not only the profound changes taking place in students as they progress through four years of medical school, but how alike they all appear at the end of those years" (1957: 25) must be qualified.

Nor are these attitudinal differences, linked to sociodemographic characteristics, erased and realigned along *intra*professional lines, such as their worksetting and specialty. Rather, differentiation and diversity in political views based on intraprofessional characteristics are added and cross-cut differences based on sociodemographic characteristics.

The difference in our findings between the effects of the religious-ethnic and socioeconomic origins of physicians on their current political ideology is critical to questions about the dynamics of socialization and social selection raised earlier in this chapter. While there is little evidence of differential social selection into medicine from the major religious-ethnic groups in the population in terms of their political views, it does seem to operate with respect to socioeconomic origins. Physicians differed only slightly, it will be recalled, in their political views according to their socioeconomic origins when they entered medical school. Moreover, whereas the religious-ethnic differences persisted, these slight socioeconomic differences faded over time. It is as though physicians, when they entered medicine, abandoned the political views, even then only dimly associated with their own socioeconomic origins. Protestant, Catholic, and Jewish physicians, on the other hand, continued to adhere to the ideology of their counterparts in the general population, perhaps because it was reinforced by their continuing identification with these groups.

Clearly, the relative effects of various sources of socialization—social and professional, early and current, continuous and discontinuous—depend, as we anticipated, on the subject matter of attitudes under examination. We have examined here only a small range of sources of socialization and types of attitudes. The study of a wider range of both "independent" variables, at more differentiated stages of the life cycle and professional career (say, precollege, premedical school, medical school, housestaff training, and professional practice), and of "dependent" variables (e.g., practitioners' orientations toward patients and various aspects of clinical style) in future inquiry is critical for a better understanding of the socialization of professionals.

More exacting methodological designs are also critical to distinguish socialization from social selection out of statuses of origin and into statuses of destination. Ideally, these questions call for longitudinal studies that would incorporate comparison samples of persons who do not become physicians drawn from strategic groups in the population, with repeated measures beginning before college or medical school, continuing at critical points throughout professional training, and extending into professional practice.

Finally, we have often alluded to the role of self-interest in influencing attitudes toward relatively specific issues. The relationship between socialization, ideology, and self-interest and their relative impact on physicians' attitudes toward specific issues remain fascinating questions for future work.

In the final chapter we discuss the implications of our findings and changes in the composition of the medical profession in forecasting its ideology in the decades ahead. It would be shortsighted, however, to argue that the future ideology of the medical profession depends solely on its composition. Its ideology is also affected by larger historical forces— broad ideological drifts in American society, the emergence and demise of specific political and health care issues, the policies and strategies adopted by organized medicine—and by differences in the thinking of distinctive *historical generations* of physicians. Our focus in the present chapter has been on physicians' social and professional characteristics, representing the influence of experiences according to their location in the social structure. In the next chapter, we turn to generational differences, representing the influence of experiences according to their location in the historical process.

Notes

1. The varying theoretical approaches are of little concern to us here since our focus is on the *content* of the norms, values, and attitudes transmitted in different socially patterned settings rather than on the *processes* and *structures* of this transmission. The range of theoretical approaches is exemplified in the chapter titles in *The Handbook of Socialization Theory and Research* (Goslin, 1969): "A Cognitive Theory of Socialization"; "Psychoanalytic Theory of Development"; "Social-Learning Theory . . ."; "Interpersonal Attraction and the Development of the Self"; "Inferences to the Socialization of the Child from Animal Studies . . ."; "Social Structure and Socialization." In an excellent review article on adult socialization, Mortimer and Simmons (1978: 429–432) distinguish among the perspectives of role theory, identification theory, generalization theory, symbolic interactionism, exchange theory, and expectancy theory.

2. On medical education, there are the classic studies by Merton, Reader, and Kendall (1957) and by Becker and others (1961) and incisive critical reviews by Bloom (1965, 1979), Fox (1973), and Light (1983). On nursing education, there is the research by Olesen and Whittaker (1968) and Simpson (1979). On dental education, the research of Sherlock and Morris (1971).

3. The relevance of individuals' nonoccupational characteristics in the study of professions is examined in: Hughes (1945: 353-359); Gouldner (1957-1958: 281-306, 444-480); Becker and Geer (1960: 304-313); Vollmer and Mills (1966: 327-355). Studies of specific occupations include the following: on business leaders, Taussig and Joslyn (1932), Warner and Abegglen (1956); on journalists, Rosten (1937) and Johnstone, Slawski, and Bowman (1976); on civil servants, Bendix (1949); on public relations men, Sussmann (1948-49: 697-708); on scientists, Knapp and Goodrich (1952); on physicians, Adams (1953: 404-409); on nurses, Hughes et al. (1958: 19-38); on the military profession, Janowitz (1960); on teachers, Colombotos (1962, 1963), and the studies cited in Havighurst and Neugarten (1967: 407-430).

4. Among these few are: on teachers, Colombotos (1962, 1963); on lawyers, Ladinsky (1963) and Carlin (1966). In a review of illustrative findings published before *The Student Physician*, Merton, Bloom, and Ramsoy (1956: 559-561), present material concerning the effects of the socioeconomic status of medical students on their use of free time and their career expectations. A monograph comparing the attitudes of medical students who are the children of physicians with those of students from other occupational backgrounds is summarized in an appendix on "Research in Progress" in *The Student Physician* (Merton, Reader, and Kendall, 1957: 298). Also, in a paper written in 1960 as these studies on medical education were drawing to a close, Kendall recognizes that characteristics of the medical student's family, such as whether his/her father was a physician and the family's socioeconomic and ethnic status, "can have profound effects on the medical student" (Kendall, 1975: 312-313). None of these findings was reported in *The Student Physician*, however, or in subsequent publications based on that project, with the exception of Kendel's dissertation that examines the effects of socioeconomic background on specialty choice versus general practice (Kendel, 1960). On the whole, Merton's study and the research that grew out of it paid little attention to the effects of social background characteristics.

5. Among these few studies are: on lawyers, Carlin (1966); on physicians, Coser (1958), Fox (1961), Seaman and Evans (1961), Kendall (1965), Gray and others (1966); Bosk (1979), Eisenberg and others (1983); and Eisenberg (1985); on teachers, Colombotos (1962).

6. Although Freidson minimizes the effects of early socialization, he does in fact introduce them to help to explain the social roots of the "clinical mentality" of practitioners. The emphasis of practitioners on autonomy and independence, he argues, stems in part from their predominantly middle-class and upper-middle-class backgrounds (1970: 170-178).

Freidson's general argument is consistent with that of the "Chicago School" in sociology that the current social situation influences behavior more than does prior socialization. But if prior professional training has little effect, why is it that we speak of the "Chicago School" in American sociology?

7. We have, of course, overdrawn the implications of Freidson's view. The imperfection of the socialization process is explicitly built into the symbolic interactionist, exchange, and expectancy theories, which view the subject as an active participant in the process. Another factor limiting the impact of any single source of socialization are the varying and potentially conflicting demands of different statuses (e.g., working class background, Protestant upbringing, psychiatric training, etc.) in the status-sets of individuals, concurrently or over time (Gross, Mason, and McEachern, 1958; Merton, 1957: 380-384).

The general question of the uniformity of the effects of socialization is forcefully raised by Dennis Wrong in a widely cited paper titled, "The oversocialized conception of man" (1961). A recent attempt to synthesize the "sociologistic" and "individualistic" orientations to socialization is found in Wentworth (1980).

8. We are not concerned here with explaining the relationship between religious affiliation or socioeconomic background or other social background characteristics, on one hand,

and the content of political ideology and other attitudes, on the other, *in the general population*—questions of long-standing interest to other researchers. Nor, as we noted earlier, are we concerned with the processes of socialization and the mechanisms by which attitudes are transmitted. These, too, have been addressed by others (see Note 1, above). We shall make only passing references to work on both of these questions.

9. The impact of "latent identities" (statuses not directly relevant to the work context) on work-related phenomena has been discussed by different authors under different labels: "dilemmas and contradictions of status" (Hughes, 1945); characteristics defining an "inner fraternity" (Hall, 1946); "latent social roles" (Gouldner, 1957, 1958; Becker and Geer, 1960); "functionally irrelevant statuses" (Merton, 1957: 380-384; Cole and Cole, 1973: 144-145).

10. Lipset and Bendix argue that upwardly mobile people in America become even more conservative than their class of destination (1964: 66-71), but the data they cite do not support their case. Maccoby and her colleagues distinguish between voting preferences and ideology: "The upward-mobile young people, while voting like their new group, retain a good part of the ideology of the group from which they came" (1954: 39).

11. In labeling health care issues as "professional" issues we are not arguing that their resolution *should* be under the sole control of the medical profession, without a lay voice. We use the term simply to refer to issues that are especially salient to the medical profession. Freidson argues that professional control should be limited not only over the *organization* of work, but over its *application* as well (1970: 335-382). Limits on professional control over the latter are exemplified in public debates over the allocation of resources to medical procedures such as renal dialysis, heroic (and costly) measures to sustain life in infants with a poor prognosis, and the like. Countering trends toward the "medicalization" of some sectors of society may be trends toward the "demedicalization," or "politicization," of others, such as the organization of medical care, and even medical practice (Fox, 1977).

12. Brim and Wheeler (1966: 24-33) list other changes in the content of early and later socialization, for example, shifts from a concern with values and motives to a concern with overt behavior; from acquisition of new material to a synthesis of the old; from a concern with idealism to a concern with realism; and from teaching expectations to teaching how to mediate conflict among expectations.

13. One could plausibly argue that attitudes play some role in "causing" certain social characteristics, say, socioeconomic status or religious affiliation (e.g., upwardly mobile minority persons may choose to become Episcopalians). But this process would apply to the *parents* of our physician respondents; it would not affect the relationship between the backgrounds of our respondents and their current attitudes.

14. The notion of "self-interest," generally implicit in social scientists' attempts to understand and explain human behavior, is most explicit in the work of economists. "Homo economicus" is graphically depicted by Adam Smith:

> Man has almost constant occasions for the help of his brethren and it is in vain for him to expect it from their *benevolence* only. He will be more likely to prevail *if he can interest their self love in his favour*, and show them that it is for their own advantage to do for him what he requires of them. It is not for the *benevolence* of the butcher, the brewer, or the baker that we can expect our dinner, *but from their regard of their own interest. (Emphasis added)*

More recently, however, social exchange theory in anthropology, sociology, and psychology has also made the concept of self-interest, under different labels, the focus of attention. (For a good review of exchange theory, see Emerson, 1981.)

In a somewhat different vein, Sears and his associates (1980) compare the effects of "self-interest" and "symbolic politics" (we prefer the terms "ideology" or "social values") on attitudes toward such diverse issues as the busing of school children, the Vietnam War, unemployment, national health insurance, and Proposition 13 in California. Although ideology has generally been found to affect attitudes toward specific issues more than does self-interest, their relative effects vary with the particular issue.

The relative effects of ideology and self-interest with respect to medical students' attitudes toward national health insurance and other issues, based on data from our 1973 national study, are being examined by Myriam Sudit.

15. These findings appear in different types of sources:

(1) Studies of voting and political behavior and of attitudes toward a range of social, political, and economic issues include the pioneering community panel surveys by Lazarsfeld and his associates, *The People's Choice*, in 1940, in Sandusky, Ohio (Lazarsfeld, Berelson, and Gaudet, 1948), and *Voting: A Study of Opinion Formation in a Presidential Campaign*, in 1948, in Elmira, New York (Berelson, Lazarsfeld, and McPhee, 1954), and the nationwide studies by a University of Michigan group (Campbell et al., 1960). (An appendix in Berelson, Lazarsfeld, and McPhee [1954: 327–347] conveniently inventories the principal findings of the major panel studies on voting up to that time.)

More wide-ranging political analyses, drawing on data from many sources, including archives of data collected by political pollsters, include the writings of Lipset (1963) and more recent analyses tracing trends in patterns of findings established by the earlier studies (Hamilton and Wright, 1975; Knoke, 1976; Abramson, 1983; and Ladd and Hadley, 1978).

More narrowly topical studies include such surveys as those on public attitudes toward NHI, which were sponsored by the American Medical Association and conducted by the Gallup organization in the late 1970s (Goodman and Steiber, 1981; Steiber and Ferber, 1981). (Lower socioeconomic groups, northeasterners, and urban dwellers are more likely than those with opposite characteristics to favor NHI in general and the more comprehensive NHI plans.)

Descriptive data produced by polling organizations such as Gallup, Louis Harris, and the New York Times/CBS News Poll as reported in the mass media also report sociodemographic differences in political attitudes.

(2) Other studies focus on an independent variable—such as religion and ethnicity (Cohn, 1958; Fuchs, 1958; and Lenski, 1961), region (Glenn and Simmons, 1967), and urban-rural differences (Glenn and Hill, 1977) in relation to a wide array of dependent variables, including political and economic-welfare attitudes.

16. Freymann (1964) saw the potential development of a "third force" in American medicine, physicians who, "with one foot firmly based on advanced training in scientific medicine and the other on private practice outside the academic sphere," may "bridge the gap" between academic and practicing physicians. Johnson argued, in 1972, that the medical associations in the United States and the United Kingdom were successful in containing divisions among segments of physicians (Johnson, 1972: 53–54).

17. Nonpractitioners—teachers, administrators, and researchers—as we noted in Chapter 3, constitute a very heterogeneous group. Their attitudes toward health care issues may well differ accordingly. Beyond that, attitudes may differ depending on specific conditions of work within each of these categories. Compare the physician-administrator in a federal health agency and one in a proprietary hospital, or the researcher at the National Institutes of Health and one in a pharmaceutical firm (on the latter, see Fox, 1961). Unfortunately, we do not have adequate numbers of cases in these various settings to make reliable statistical comparisons.

18. Some specialties within the broadly defined "surgical" and "medical" groupings do in fact overlap in prestige—cardiology, a medical specialty, is second only to thoracic surgery and neurosurgery, and higher in prestige level than the other surgical specialties (Shortell, 1974: 4). But the pattern we have just described generally holds.

19. In contrast to this line of reasoning, however, studies of American academics have shown that it is those professors at the elite universities, at the higher professional ranks, and those who are more satisfied professionally who hold more liberal opinions (Ladd and Lipset, 1975). The relationship of satisfaction to political views is certainly more complex than is implied here; it depends on the sources and objects of satisfaction and on their perceived relationship to specific political issues (see Lipset and Schwartz, 1966).

20. This dimension in the patient-practitioner relationship has been conceptualized in slightly different ways and used in different types of empirical investigations: Szasz and Hollander (1956); Freidson (1960); Bynder (1965); Gray and others (1966); Shortell (1974).

21. A more precise test of this reasoning would require characterizing physicians according to the attitudes of *their* patients, or, more realistically, according to, say, a proxy measure, such as the socioeconomic composition of their patient loads.

22. An example used to illustrate the effects of social context is the influence of the socioeconomic composition of students in a high school on college plans: controlling for individual students' socioeconomic status, students in high SES schools are more likely than those in low SES schools to go to college.

23. The general idea that values inherent in different professions are associated with different political ideologies is suggested by Michels, Durkheim, Mannheim, and Laski (cited and discussed in Lipset and Schwartz, 1966: 308). See also Ladd and Lipset, 1975: 55–124, for a discussion of differences among the political views of faculty in different disciplines. Lipset and Schwartz note, as examples, the questioning nature of the scientist's mind and the lawyer's and historian's concern with the past, associated with liberal and conservative political views, respectively. The rationale can easily be extended to specialties within professions, or even to schools of thought within specialties. Within psychiatry, for example, those with an analytic and psychological orientation tended to be more liberal in their attitudes toward Medicare than those with a directive and organic orientation (Colombotos, 1968: 330).

24. It should be noted with respect to the slight differences among the four major regions, that we found much stronger inter- and intrastate differences in physicians' attitudes. For example, the proportion of physicians who favored "some form" of national health insurance ranges from highs of 73 percent in Massachusetts and 71 percent in Maryland to lows of 25 percent in Mississippi and 33 percent in South Carolina; and, in 1964, 48 percent of New York City practitioners favored Medicare, compared with only 20 percent of upstate New York practitioners (Colombotos, Kirchner, and Millman, 1975b; Colombotos, 1968).

25. See, for example, our earlier studies based on the responses of New York State private practitioners in the sixties (Colombotos, 1968, 1969d, 1971); a national study of office-based general practitioners, internists, pediatricians, and obstetricians in the early seventies (Mechanic, 1974); and a study of Yale University medical graduates based on several questions from our 1973 national study (Goldman, 1974a,b). In a study of physicians in the Detroit area, Heins found, as we did, that women physicians were more liberal politically than men (1979: 230–232). Other surveys of physicians' attitudes include those done regularly since the seventies by the American Medical Association, occasional surveys by such magazines as the *Medical World News, Medical Economics,* and the *Medical Tribune,* and special surveys such as those done by Louis Harris for the Kaiser Foundation and the Equitable Life Assurance Society (Louis Harris and Associates, 1981, 1983, 1984).

26. For a concise description of hierarchical multiple regression, see Nie and others, *Statistical Package for the Social Sciences,* 1975: 337–340, 344–345.

27. See note 19.

28. A closer look at the beta's ("path coefficients" in a path analysis) connecting physi-

cians' socioeconomic background, their *fathers'* political party preferences, their own *early* political party preferences and their *current* political party preferences reveals a complex picture. Physicians from upper socioeconomic backgrounds were only slightly more likely than those from lower socioeconomic backgrounds to consider themselves Republicans when they *started medical school.* This is explained by the influence of their *fathers'* party preferences. Controlling for their fathers' party preferences and their own early party preferences, however, physicians' socioeconomic background had a slight, though statistically nonsignificant, *negative* influence on their *current* political ideology and party preferences (beta's were $-.04$ and $-.03$, respectively). That is, physicians from upper socioeconomic backgrounds were slightly more liberal than those from lower socioeconomic backgrounds.

A clue for interpreting this pattern of results is provided by noting that, although the *fathers'* party preferences strongly influenced the *early* party preferences of their physician-children and the physicians' *early* preferences strongly influenced their *current* preferences, the *direct* effect of the fathers' preferences on the current preferences of physicians, after controlling for physicians' early preferences as an intervening variable, was negative! That is to say, among physicians who were *early Democrats,* those with Republican fathers were *more* likely than those with Democratic fathers to be *current Democrats*; among physicians who were *early Republicans,* the same. In short, *early rebels* were *less* likely to end up in the same political camp as their fathers than *early conformists.* To do so would mean to switch their party preferences twice.

In the earlier New York State study, it should be noted, physicians' socioeconomic background was also only barely related to both their fathers' and their own early and current political views (Colombotos, 1969d).

29. Physicians' emphasis on professional autonomy influenced their attitudes, especially those toward health care issues, partially through the worksettings of physicians (the more they emphasized autonomy, the less likely they were to be in organized settings), but also directly. Autonomy, in turn, was influenced only by the gender of physicians: men emphasized it slightly more.

30. Mechanic also found that physicians' general dissatisfaction was related to their acceptance of changes in the organization of health care (1974).

31. Some qualifying remarks should be attached to these findings:

(1) The accuracy of physicians' recall of their political party preferences when they "started medical school" is open to question. If they have a tendency to respond so that their early preferences are consistent with their current preferences, then this pattern would overestimate the selection argument; if inconsistent, the socialization argument. The former is more plausible than the latter, we would argue.

(2) Medical students' career *plans* do not always materialize. The attenuated relationship between plans and attitudes would thus tend to underestimate the amount of selection into professional statuses. We limited our analysis to *fourth-year* students, who are more likely to be certain about their plans than their younger classmates, in order to minimize this effect.

Given the limitations of cross-sectional designs with respect to distinguishing between selection and socialization to explain statistical asssociations, it is not surprising that arguments for either are based on the appeal of plausibility and on usually weak supporting data. Wolinsky, for example, argues that the relationships he found between physicians' practice settings and career attitudes in a cross-sectional study are due to selection (1982: 415).

5 Generational Differences in American Medicine

In the late 1960s and early 1970s a much publicized "new breed" of physician entered the nation's medical schools. Compared with their professional elders, they were characterized as being more liberal politically, more committed to reforming the health care system to meet people's needs, more egalitarian in their relationships with patients and other health practitioners, and less competitive and less driven in their work (see "Unrest on the medical campus," 1967; Lewis, 1969a, b; "Medical students: Healers become activists," 1969; "Medicine's own generation gap," 1969; "Today's young doctor looks at medicine," 1971; Farnsworth, 1970; "The new doctor . . . ," 1972; Fox, 1973; Funkenstein, 1978: 12–13, 22–26, 54–55). This change was a part of the political and cultural movements that swept the nation's colleges and universities during this period (civil rights, the war in Southeast Asia, and university reform) bringing dramatic shifts in students' attitudes toward politics, work, marriage and the family, and the role of women (Yankelovich, 1972; Braungart, 1980).

It was debated even then whether that sharp break between the younger and older medical generations would continue into the future. Would students entering medical school in the seventies and eighties share the views of those who had entered in the late sixties? Would the attitudes of students who entered medicine during the sixties persist over their lives, thereby transforming the ideology of the medical profession? (See "A second look at last year's radicals," 1970; Goldman and Ebbert, 1973; Lewis and Winer, 1976; Coe, Pepper, and Mattis, 1977; Funkenstein, 1978; and, with respect to college youth, see Braungart, 1980).

The new breed of medical student is less visible today than a decade ago. This may be because today's medical students are more similar to the pre-sixties generation. A more likely explanation is that although the political activism and confrontation tactics of the sixties are less in vogue today, some significant, basic attitudes of the medical students of that era continue to characterize today's medical students. They are still "socially concerned . . . critical of the way health care is organized . . . determined to practice a more equitable, feeling, and less driven medicine than [their] elders . . . , reluctant to accept the "on-call 24 hours a day demands" [associated with] many branches of traditional practice . . . staunchly egalitarian in [their] conception of the doctor, the doctor's relationship to patients, and to nonphysician members of the medical team" (Fox, 1973: 211, 217). (In a recent personal communication, Fox speculated that her profile still applied in the eighties.)

Less visible and dramatic, but, we would argue, perhaps more significant than the "generation gap" between medical students and physicians in the late 1960s, were differences in the thinking of physicians who entered medicine at different times in the decades preceding the sixties. Approximately a fourth of the country's physicians in 1973 had entered medicine before the end of World War II; approximately 10 percent had entered after the passage of Medicare in 1965. The interval between these periods saw sweeping changes in the organization of health care—for example, in the role of government, the organization of medical practice, and methods of reimbursement and payment, which we discussed in Chapter 2.

In this chapter we compare the attitudes of medical students and housestaff toward political and health care issues according to their year in training and the attitudes of senior physicians according to their age. Observed differences can be interpreted in two ways: they may be due to either historical-generational differences or to aging or life-cycle changes. The distinction is important, for the two explanations point to different sources of socialization: in the *generation* case, to the influence of historical events; in the *life-cycle* case, to the influence of professional training, career stage, and other sources associated with life cycle. This distinction is also important for forecasting the future thinking of the profession as a whole.

If younger and older physicians differ in their attitudes and the younger hold on to their attitudes as they move through life, the attitudinal profile of the profession is transformed as the older physicians retire. If, as they age, the younger physicians become like older physicians in their thinking, the picture is more stable. Retiring elderly conservatives, for example, are replaced by physicians who become, in their turn, as conservative as their predecessors.

One-time cross-sectional data such as ours cannot resolve this question. We therefore exploit other sources—data from other studies, including generational-cohort data (we use the terms "generation" and "cohort" interchangeably, though, as we explain below, we prefer "generation"); "recall" data from our 1973 respondents about their political party preference when they started medical school; and various kinds of "side information" (a term coined by Converse, 1976: 20–24), such as our knowledge about historical events and trends, professional training settings, and careers. We turn to all these sources in order to make a plausible case for generational differences or life-cycle changes with respect to various patterns of findings.[1]

Before presenting our data, we want to expand a bit on the concepts of "generation," "cohort," and "period" effects, to show how they provide a rationale for our analysis.

Conceptual and Methodological Issues: Generations, Cohorts, and Periods

In his classical formulation, Mannheim (1952: 291) compared a generation to a social class as follows:

> The fact of belonging to the same class, and that of belonging to the same generation or age group, have this in common, that both endow the individuals sharing in them with a common location in the social and *historical process*, and thereby limit them to a specific range of potential *experience*, predisposing them for a *certain characteristic mode of thought and experience*, and a characteristic type of historically relevant action. (*Emphasis added*)

Central to Mannheim's formulation is the unique constellation of historical experiences that characterizes a generation. We shall return to this point below because it underlies potential confusion between "generation" and "period."

In an influential paper, Ryder (1965) explicated the relationship between cohort differences and social change through "demographic metabolism." The concept of political generation has informed the analysis of political ideology and political party preference in the United States and elsewhere (Heberle, 1951; Hyman, 1959: 123–154; Campbell et al., 1960; Abramson, 1975, 1983; Converse, 1976). A plethora of research on adolescents and the elderly draws heavily on the concept, spurred, in the first case, by the campus activism of the sixties, and in the second, by concern about the needs and consequencs of the swelling number of elderly in our society. (On the younger generation, see Braungart, 1980; Elder, 1980; on the older generation, see Riley, Johnson, and Foner, 1972;

Bengtson and Cutler, 1976; Hudson and Binstock, 1976). This substantive research has in turn spawned considerable work on conceptual and methodological issues (Elder, 1975; Bengtson and Cutler, 1976; Glenn, 1977; Kertzer, 1983), including attempts to differentiate "generation," "cohort," "period," and "aging" (see Note 1).

The terms "generation" and "cohort" are technically equivalent. The former is generally used by sociologists and historians in the Mannheimian tradition, and the latter, by demographers (Ryder, 1965: 844–845). Both are defined as "those people within a geographically or otherwise delineated population who experienced the same significant life event within a given period of time" (Glenn, 1977: 8). In demography, the "significant life event" is usually birth, hence the term "birth cohort."

But the two terms differ in nuance. "The crux of Mannheim's concept of generation . . . ," Bengtson and Cutler note "lies in its intermingling of birth-cohort categories, historical experience, and political consciousness" (1976: 136). Many social scientists "have emptied the concept of generation of its active political meaning . . . and have treated generational location simply in birth-cohort terms." A pity, we would add. In this chapter we use the term "generation" in this historical and political sense.[2]

People can be classified according to life events other than birth. In our analysis we think of medical students and housestaff according to when they entered college and medical school, and senior physicians according to when they entered medical school and entered practice. These stages can be more or less accurately defined in terms of each other. Most physicians begin medical school in their early twenties, graduate in their mid-twenties, and enter practice in their late twenties or early thirties (although older physicians, who are not as likely to have taken residency training, may have entered practice a little younger). We then ask, at what point in their lives are the attitudes of physicians most affected by historical events? This question is critical for a close analysis of the influence of the events of the late sixties and early seventies on the attitudes of medical students and housestaff. It is less critical in analyzing the effects of incremental trends on the attitudes of senior physicians in previous decades.

"Generational effects," that is, differences between generations attributable to their unique combinations of experiences, are distinguished from "period effects," the influence of specific events on people of all ages. Whereas members of different generations may all be exposed to some of the same historical events (e.g., physicians just entering practice and those about to leave it were both exposed to the passage and implementation of Medicare in the mid-sixties), each generation differs from all others with respect to the *combination* of events to which its members have been exposed.

The influence of a given event (a "period effect"), moreover, is likely to vary among different generations since specific past experiences may blunt or accentuate, or otherwise modify, the effects of that event. Non-historical factors may also affect the way different age groups experience an event. Older people are commonly viewed as more rigid in their ways than younger people; the impact of new events may be blunted by the mere number of previous experiences.[3] The association of different roles and statuses with age may also modify the effects of a given event on different generations. Older physicians close to retirement might respond quite differently from younger physicians, for example, to a national health insurance plan with strict controls on the income of physicians.

Period influences, in brief, are likely to interact with generational and age differences rather than simply to add to them. This empirical blurring of "generation" and "period" prompts Converse to refer to them as one-and-a-half, rather than as two, distinct classes of effects (Converse, 1976: 18–24; see also Glenn, 1977: 52–53, 59–60).

We want to link the attitudes of students, housestaff, and physicians toward political and health care issues in 1973 to two separate sets of historical events: first to the dramatic and tumultuous movements of the late sixties that focused on civil rights, the war in Southeast Asia, and university reform, all of which spilled over onto medical school campuses and into issues concerning the delivery of health care; and second to the less visible and slower-moving trends in political thinking and the organization of health care in the decades before that, extending back into the thirties.

Our classification of generations among medical students and housestaffs on the one hand, and physicians, on the other, reflects differences in the content and tempo of these two sets of events and our conception of their differential impact on these two *sets* of generations. Because we view the relevant events in the decades preceding the sixties as incremental trends rather than as sharply defined dramatic events, it is not as critical to divide our senior physicians into annual cohorts in which a "significant life event" (say entry into medical school or practice) is tagged to a specific historical event within a circumscribed time period.

Thus, in our tabular analysis, we divide students and housestaff into annual cohorts in order to register the impact of the fast-moving events of the late sixties and early seventies; we classify senior physicians into ten-year cohorts, beginning with those 35 or under and ending with those 65 or over.[4]

Figure 5-1a portrays the calendar years of "professional life events"—

Figure 5–1a. Historical Periods Corresponding to Significant Life Events (College, Medical School, Housestaff Training) of 1973 Cohorts of Medical Students and Housestaff

1961 1962 1963 1964 1965 1966 1967 1968 1969 1970 1971 1972 1973	Cohorts in 1973
	Medical students
OOOOOOOOOOOOOOOO---------	1st year
OOOOOOOOOOOOOOOO-----------------	2nd year
OOOOOOOOOOOOOOOO-----------------------	3rd year
OOOOOOOOOOOOOOOO-----------------------------	4th year
	Housestaff
OOOOOOOOOOOOOOOO---------------------------XXXXX	1st year
OOOOOOOOOOOOOOOO---------------------------XXXXXXXXX	2nd year
OOOOOOOOOOOOOOOO---------------------------XXXXXXXXXXXXX	3rd year
OOOOOOOOOOOOOOOO---------------------------XXXXXXXXXXXXXXXXX	4th year
OOOOOOOOOOOOOOOO---------------------------XXXXXXXXXXXXXXXXXXXXX	5th year

OOOOO In college
----- In medical school
XXXXX In housestaff training

entry and graduation from college and medical school—of the medical student and housestaff cohorts in our study in the Spring of 1973. Figure 5-1b does the same for senior physicians, fixing entry to medical school and practice according to decade. These help to link the professional and personal lives of our generations to historical events and thereby to develop a rationale for predicting the impact of these events on their thinking in 1973.

Two components enter into developing such a rationale: first, locating specific events more precisely in time and considering their potential impact on medical students, housestaff, and senior physicians as an aggregate, and second, identifying those points in the lives of medical students, housestaff, and senior physicians when a given event is likely to have the greatest impact on their thinking.

With respect to the first issue, although there were stirrings on college and medical school campuses in the mid-sixties, these movements peaked in 1968-70.[5] In 1970, as a result of the invasion of Cambodia and the killings at Kent State and Jackson State, 57 percent of the nation's colleges experienced protests that had a "significant impact" on campus operations (Braungart, 1980: 566). In 1968, medical students took over the deans' meeting at the Association of American Medical Colleges, and in 1969, they demonstrated at the AMA convention ("Today's young doctor looks at medicine," 1971).

Figure 5–1b. Historical Periods Corresponding to When 1973 Cohorts of Senior Physicians Were in Practice

1920	1925	1930	1935	1940	1945	1950	1955	1960	1965	1973	Age in 1973
									xxxxxxxxxx-----		Under 35
								xxxxxxxxxx--------------			35–44
						xxxxxxxxxx---------------------------------					45–54
				xxxxxxxxxx---							55–64
		xxxxxxxxxx---										65 or over

xxxxx In medical school and housestaff training (midpoint for each generation-cohort)

----- In practice (midpoint for each generation cohort, assuming physician entered practice at age 30)

It should be noted that the events of the late sixties may not have had equal impact on the attitudes of medical students and housestaff toward *all* of the political and health care issues that are the focus of our analysis. We suspect, for example, that the effect was greater on attitudes toward issues linked to general political ideology, governmental responsibility for providing adequate medical care (spurred by events and thinking originating outside academic medical centers), and the provision and accessibility of medical care than on attitudes toward peer reviews.

There is little evidence or theory as a basis for addressing the question: which of our trainee-generations in 1973, because of their being at different stages in their lives in the late 1960s and early 1970s, were most impressed by these events? Our youngest trainees entered college in the fall of 1968 while the oldest had graduated from medical school by June of 1968, a few months earlier. Anecdotal evidence suggests that in 1969 it was those medical students in their first and second years who were the most active (Lewis, 1969a: 67, 70; "Medicine's own generation gap," 1969: 23). Another study suggests that the "primary" leaders were drawn mainly from the second and third years (Lewis, 1969b: 1031).

It is plausible to assume that: (1) the impact of the events from the late sixties to the early seventies increased, incrementally and cumulatively, during this period, through 1973; and (2) this increasing overall impact had a stronger effect on the younger generations, because of their relatively greater impressionability, than on the older generations. If these assumptions are correct, then we would find that the younger generations among medical students and housestaff hold more liberal views than do the older generations.

The events of the sixties, we reasoned, had less impact on senior physicians as a group than on physicians in training and little impact among senior physicians according to their generation. Conversely, except for the most advanced housestaff, trainees either were not exposed to or did not meaningfully experience the decades prior to the sixties. Freshman medical students in 1973, it should be noted, entered college in 1968; the most advanced housestaff, before 1960. Senior physicians, on the other hand, did experience the pre-sixties. We assumed, moreover, that the earlier they entered medical school or practice, during the early development of trends in health care (discussed in Chapter 2), the more likely they were to resist subsequent expansion of these developments, that is, the more likely they were to resist subsequent "period" influences. If we are correct, then we should find that, as of 1973, older physicians were more likely than younger physicians to have conservative views toward these issues.

Findings

Description of Findings

Three broad patterns emerge in the attitudes of medical student, housestaff, and senior physician generations (Table 5-1).

First, with respect to their attitudes toward political and government-in-medicine issues, there were sharp, incremental, and consistent differences among students and housestaff according to their year in training—the more advanced taking more conservative positions than those in earlier stages on each of these issues.[6]

In contrast, among senior physicians, although the younger were a bit more likely than the older to hold liberal views, the differences were much smaller and not consistently incremental. The large difference in liberal attitudes over the nine-plus-year interval bounded by first-year medical students and advanced housestaff is all the more remarkable when compared with the smaller difference over the 30-plus-year interval bounded by those senior physicians under 35 and those 65 or over.

Second, the pattern of attitudes toward the two "financial" health care issues was somewhat similar to that for political and government-in-medicine attitudes. Support for both salaried and/or capitation payment and for prepayment declined with year in training among students and housestaff, though the drop was not as sharp as it was with respect to political and government-in-medicine issues, nor was it strictly decremental; and it levelled off among senior physicians according to their age.

Third, in contrast, attitudes toward the three more "organizational" issues—group practice, peer reviews, and the delegation of tasks—showed

Table 5-1. Generational Differences in Attitudes Toward Political and Health Care Issues[a]

	Base N's	Political ideology (% liberal)	Gov't. in medicine (% liberal)	Group practice scale (% favor)	Peer review (% favor)	Task delegation (% favor)	Physician reimbursement: Salaried/capitation (% accept)	Prepayment (% accept)
Medical students								
First year	925	77	74	36	48	39	45	61
Second year	902	73	69	44	50	34	41	58
Third year	818	68	69	44	51	41	36	54
Fourth year	769	64	66	49	52	43	38	57
USMG housestaff								
First year	207	61	61	58	50	53	40	54
Second year	168	58	61	55	55	54	36	56
Third year	163	54	52	49	55	54	28	43
Fourth year	147	52	60	44	48	52	21	48
Fifth or more year	168	38	42	45	51	54	23	49
r =		.22	.15	.09	—	-.11	.13	.07
Senior physicians								
Under 35	306	51	54	50	55	55	34	49
35–44	847	42	47	42	46	46	29	42
45–54	785	37	42	34	37	41	30	40
55–64	527	34	43	34	33	32	27	41
65 or over	248	40	48	25	20	27	33	44
r =		.07	.07	.17	.20	.20	—	.04

[a]See notes to Table 4-1.

an opposite pattern: here, the attitudes of medical students and housestaff fluctuated according to their year in training, whereas support by senior physicians on all three issues dropped sharply and consistently according to their age.

Medical students and housestaff barely differed in their attitudes toward peer reviews according to their year in training; housestaff, as a group, were a bit more favorable than medical students, as a group, toward the delegation of tasks, but neither group differed among themselves according to their year in training.

The attitudes of students and housestaff toward group practice were different—and puzzling. As measured by a scale of three questions (perception of which practice arrangement led to the "best medical care"; which arrangement, assuming "your income in all of these were the same," was "most desirable"; and which one was "least desirable"—see section on "Measures and Scales" in the Appendix), there was a curvilinear relationship between attitudes toward group practice and year-in-training: support for group practice peaked among first-year housestaff.

Although the three items were highly intercorrelated, an examination of the generations' responses to each of the three questions reveals a differentiated picture. It turns out that the curvilinear relationship between year of training and the scale of attitudes toward group practice is accounted for solely by their responses to the question asking about the most "undesirable" form of practice. "Solo practice" was least popular among first-year housestaff; 70 percent considered it the most undesirable, "rising" from 36 percent of first-year medical students and "dropping" to 58 percent among housestaff beyond their fourth year of training. Conversely, in a nearly mirror-image pattern, opposition to the two "large group" practice options was lowest among these same first-year housestaff.

Trainees' attitudes toward the more organized forms of practice as indicated by their perceptions of which arrangement led to the "best medical care" and which arrangement was "most desirable" were generally more positive according to year in training, whereas, as we just noted, the attitudes of senior physicians on all three items in the scale were more negative according to their age.[7]

Discussion and Interpretation of Findings

What are we to make of these findings? Do attitudinal differences, where they exist, between career-stage and age-generations reflect life-cycle (aging) or generational-period influences?

Political and Government-in-Medicine Issues

We were surprised to find that among senior physicians the younger were only slightly more liberal than the older in their political and government-in-medicine views.

Other studies of the political and government-in-medicine views of physicians, however, have shown similar results. Surveys of physicians in the 1930s "showed no major differences of opinion between the age groups" toward "medical-economic" issues (Garceau, 1941: 133); in 1955, there were essentially no age differences among physicians in their views toward the role of government in the field of health (National Opinion Research Center, undated). More recent surveys generally yield the same findings: physicians differ little, if at all, in their attitudes toward these issues according to their age (Louis Harris and Associates, 1984).

Among physicians in our study, there was a slight net shift in their preferences from the Democratic party and toward the Republican since starting medical school. Moreover, the older they were, the more likely they were to have made this shift (except for those 65 or over, who were no more likely to have shifted than those under 35). But, age differences in relation to their political party preference "when [they] started medical school" were quite similar to those in relation to their present preferences.

These lines of analysis, however, provide no substantial clue as to why age differences in the political and government-in-medicine views of physicians are smaller than age differences in the general population.[8] One speculation is that because the medical profession may "select" potentially conservative people from all groups in society, the range of political opinion within which physicians may differ according to generational, period, or aging influences is limited. This explanation does not, however, fit with the finding of sizeable differences in the political views of physicians according to other social and professional characteristics, such as their religious background and worksetting, as we showed in Chapter 4.

Turning our attention to students and housestaffs, what most plausibly explains the strong differences in their political and government-in-medicine views—generational, period, or aging influences? Data from other studies are helpful. One source is a continuing series of surveys of California medical students and recent graduates conducted by the California Medical Association at three-year intervals between 1969 and 1981 inquiring about several issues similar to ours (California Medical Association, 1982). A second source is a study based on interviews with freshman medical students each year between 1970 and 1975 and with seniors in 1974 and 1975 at the St. Louis University School of Medicine (Coe et al., 1977).

Both studies show an increasing liberalism among freshman medical students, and, in the California surveys, among students and housestaff at each stage of training, up to 1972, with respect to government participation in financing and changing the organization of medical care. In both studies, this pattern was followed by conservative shifts after 1972.

This turning point, the early and mid-seventies, it will be recalled, corresponds roughly to Funkenstein's demarcation between the "Student Activism Era" (1969–70) and the "Doldrums Era" (1971–74) in medical schools (1978: 11–14); to politically conservative shifts among college youth between 1971 and 1975 (see Braungart, 1980: 576–577); and to the beginning of disenchantment with liberal reform and Great Society programs (Starr, 1982: 379–419).

The pattern is best exemplified by the data from the California study in Table 5-2. First-year students, fourth-year students, and graduates from three years earlier all took more liberal positions in 1972 than their counterparts in 1969. Reading across the columns, one finds that 43 percent of the freshman medical students took a liberal position in 1972, compared with 29 percent of those in 1969; 40 percent of the seniors took a liberal position in 1972, compared with 24 percent of these in 1969; 36 percent of the three-year graduates took a liberal position in 1972, compared with 17 percent of those in 1969.

Table 5–2. California Medical Students' and Graduates' Attitudes Toward the Role of Government in Medical Practice[a] by Period and Cohort

	1969	1972	1975	1978	1981
First-year medical students	29[b]	43	35	26	28
	(185)	(198)	(248)	(265)	(244)
Fourth-year medical students	24	40	29	26	21
	(137)	(120)	(114)	(158)	(178)
Three-year graduates	17	36	27	10	20
	(92)	(99)	(64)	(90)	(99)
Six-year graduates	—	25	19	—	11
		(73)	(47)		(64)
Ten-year graduates	—		18	—	—
			(50)		

[a]The question was: "It seems only reasonable that government should have a strong voice in determining the organizational form of medical practice through which medical services are provided."

[b]Figures outside parentheses are percentages of each group who agree with the statement, a "liberal" response; figures in parentheses are the total number of each group.

Source: California Medical Association, 1982.

The political winds shifted, however, between 1972 and 1975. Students and graduates at each stage were more conservative in 1975 than in 1972: 35 percent of the freshmen were liberal in 1975 compared with 43 percent in 1972; and so on.

Clearly, "period" effects were operating during these intervals. Together with our findings showing that in 1973 the younger cohorts were much more liberal in their thinking on a range of political and government-in-medicine issues (see Table 5-1) than the older cohorts, the liberal shift from 1969 to 1972 is also compatible with our assumption that the younger cohorts would be more influenced than the older cohorts by events during the late sixties and early seventies.

But this assumption is not supported if we take a closer look at the California Medical Association data in Table 5-2. We note that the *intra*cohort liberal changes from 1969-72, consistent with the general liberal "period" change during this interval, were no larger for the younger cohorts than for the older ones. Reading diagonally, 29 percent of the 1969 freshmen were liberal in 1969; 40 percent, as seniors, in 1972 (a difference of 11%). Twenty-four percent of the 1969 seniors were liberal in 1969; 36 percent, three years out of medical school, in 1972 (a difference of 12%). Seventeen percent of the 1969 third-year housestaffs were liberal in 1969; 25 percent, three years later, in 1972 (a difference of 8%). We note also that the size of the *intra*cohort changes in the opposite direction after 1972, consistent with the general conservative "period" change, did not differ among the cohorts.

If younger trainees were more impressed than the older trainees by the conservative period shift in the mid-seventies and late seventies, then the differences between the political thinking of younger and older trainees in the late seventies and early eighties (the column percentages in Table 5-2) would be flattened out. That was not the case. Although the overall level of liberal-conservative attitudes varied from period to period, younger trainees were consistently more liberal than their elder classmates.[9] These data suggest the *additive* effects of period and aging influences.[10]

Health Care Issues

We are quite comfortable with the plausibility of attributing the major portion of the variation in the attitudes of *senior physicians* toward group practice, peer reviews, and task delegation to generational influences rather than to career-stage-age effects. Physicians entering medical practice when these trends were well underway were more likely to accept them, we argued, than physicians who entered practice earlier; the latter were more likely to resist changes in a style of practice to which they had already become accustomed.

This explanation is supported by comparing our data with those from a study conducted in 1955 (National Opinion Research Center, undated). Within each age group, physicians in 1973 were much more likely than those in 1955 to prefer the more organized forms of practice (Table 5-3).[11] Here, too, however, these data, like the trainee data in the California study, *could* be due to the additive effects of period and aging influences. But here, the generational, or period-interaction-with-age, explanation seems to us more plausible. There is no apparent reason why physicians should become more resistant to group practice, peer reviews, and task-delegation as they grow older.

It is always difficult—and challenging to the analyst's creativity—to explain data that do not support his or her hypotheses. The absence of age differences in the attitudes of physicians toward salaried/capitation practice and prepayment, we might speculate, may be due to the neutralizing effects of two sets of influences. Younger physicians may be more likely than their older colleagues to accept these trends because of generational and period influences, while older physicians may be more likely than younger physicians to accept them as an income cushion as they begin to cut down on their practice.[12] Ideology and self-interest neutralize each other.

Accounting for the attitudes of *medical students* and *housestaff* toward health care issues according to their year in training is also difficult. The differences, where they exist, were not as strong or as consistent as those with respect to their attitudes toward political and government-in-medi-

Table 5-3. Percentage of Physicians Choosing "Individual" ("Solo") Practice as "Most Desirable" by Age in 1955 and 1973

	1955[a]	1973[b]
39 or under	29 (122)	6 (694)
40–49	36 (165)	13 (828)
50–59	47 (110)	14 (653)
60 or over	64 (71)	25 (540)

[a]National Opinion Research Center, (Q. 79B), undated.
[b]1973 national sample.

cine issues. The best we can do is to offer some ad hoc interpretations of some of these relationships.

If we assume that period influences interact with year-in-training, the younger being more impressionable than the older, the *increase* in the desirability of group practice[13] and, to a lesser extent, task delegation according to year-in-training flies in the face of influences making group practice and task delegation more acceptable during the late 1960s and early 1970s. This pattern, therefore, is likely to be due to individual changes in the attitudes of students and housestaff as they move through their training. Perhaps it is the continued exposure of trainees to situations in which medical care is highly institutionalized and characterized by a highly complex division of labor that "socializes" trainees toward increasing acceptance of "group practice" and "task delegation." Or, it is plausible that generational/period influences operated in interaction with career stage, but counter to the pattern we assumed earlier, namely, that the young tend to be more responsive than the old to period changes. In this case, period changes may have "taken hold" more among those further along in their training, possibly because the choice of type of practice arrangement was more imminent and salient and better informed among them than it was among early trainees.

Apparently, however, the attitudes of trainees toward peer reviews, which also characterize their training settings, were not affected. Or, this apparent stability could be the net result of two opposing and neutralizing, trends: (1) an increasing self-confidence in trainees as they proceed through their training (Bucher and Stelling observe that by the time they have finished their training, their self-confidence has burgeoned [1977: 282]), which makes them more accepting of peer reviews; and (2) continuing supervision in the face of this increasing self-confidence, which make them more negative.

Summary

Our findings indicate that the sweeping assertions about a "new breed" of physician entering the nation's medical schools in the late sixties and early seventies should be qualified.

The "generation gap" between student physicians and their professional elders in 1973 was not as sharply defined nor did it extend to as wide a range of issues as was publicized. The gap appears to have been limited primarily to political and government-in-medicine issues. Moreover, the shift toward liberal views was a temporary "period" effect affecting all trainees. By the mid-seventies, the political winds had shifted rightward, and so had the political views of students and housestaffs. Moreover, the weaker liberal views of advanced trainees compared with those of early trainees appear to be due more to individual changes than to the greater impressionability of younger trainees to the larger political environment, as we had hypothesized. These "changes" tapered off as housestaff entered practice: the political views of advanced housestaff (with the exception of those in their fifth year of training or beyond, who were mainly in surgical residencies) differed little from those of young physicians in practice, and young physicians differed little from older physicians.

The turbulent events of the sixties obscured the impact of less visible and more glacierlike, but potentially more significant and enduring, changes in the organization of health care in the decades preceding the sixties, changes that have left their mark on the views of successive, more broadly defined generations of physicians. Those who entered practice after the passage of Medicare were much more willing than those who entered before World War II to accept group practice, peer reviews, and the delegation of tasks. These sharp, linear differences, which we interpret as generational differences, overshadowed any patterned differences in the attitudes of students and housestaff toward health care issues according to their year in training. Where the latter did occur (e.g., more favorable attitudes toward group practice and task delegation and less favorable attitudes toward salaried reimbursement and prepayment among advanced trainees than among early trainees), they are more plausibly attributed to individual changes than to generational or period influences. In any case, the views of advanced housestaff, again, seemed to merge closely with the views of young physicians in practice.

Describing our findings is one thing; explaining them is another. Whether observed differences represent generational, period, or career-stage-age influences is, as we noted earlier, problematic, especially in cross-sectional studies such as ours with an occasional introduction of cohort data from other studies. We have speculated freely on the meaning of these data, often resting our case on the appeal of plausibility.

Beyond issuing the conventional cautionary note, however, we want to bring attention to some substantive and methodological points inherent in the data and the analysis. It is possible that the headline-making events that characterized the late sixties on our medical campuses and teaching hospitals had little relevance to the health care issues under examination here: group practice, peer reviews, task delegation, salaried reimbursement, and prepayment. Moreover, it is possible that our differentiating generations of trainees according to their year in training was too narrow to register the volatile events of the sixties (under the assumption that younger, early trainees were more impressionable than older, advanced trainees). More broadly defined generations may have been more appropriate. The conceptual and temporal delineation of both historical events and generations is critical in establishing linkages between them. With these considerations in mind, the case for generational and period-interacting-with-age-or-career-stage influences to explain attitudinal differences among students and housestaffs according to year in training is weakened; it is more plausible to explain these differences as individual changes.

Whether differences between "generations" of trainees and physicians are due, indeed, to generational, period, or aging influences will affect the ideological makeup of the profession in the decades that follow. We discuss these implications in our concluding chapter, drawing on findings discussed in this chapter as well as on the results of studies conducted since the mid-seventies.

But forecasts of the ideology of the profession should anticipate and take into account future events that may affect the thinking of physicians. These future events may be viewed as "period" influences. We turn, in the next chapter, to a detailed examination of how physicians responded to one such event, a major and dramatic event, in the past: the passage and implementation of Medicare.

Notes

1. Even cohort analysis, repeated measurements of two or more cohorts at two or more points in time, cannot conclusively separate the effects of "generation-cohort," "period," and "aging" since each variable is a function of the other two. (See Converse, 1976: 20; Glenn, 1977: 13–14. For an attempt to unravel these effects by assuming their additivity rather than their interaction, see Mason et al., 1973; and for a debate on this issue, see Glenn, 1977: 59; Rodgers, 1982; and Smith, Mason, and Fienberg, 1982.)

2. Some formulations of "cohort" include social characteristics, such as level of education, as components of the concept (see Ryder, 1965; Elder, 1975: 168, fn. 4). Our emphasis is on the undifferentiated effects of social historical events and experiences on the thinking of whole generations of physicians. To the extent that generation units, "groups within the same actual generation which work up the material of their common experience in different specific ways" (Mannheim, 1952: 304), are based on sociodemographic characteristics, one may conceive of differentiated effects of general historical events on such subgroups within the society (see, e.g., Brunswick, 1970), or in our case, within the medical profession.

3. Older persons, however, are not necessarily less affected by events than younger persons. An economic depression and unemployment may have a stronger and more lasting impact on adult breadwinners, for example, than on adolescents (Hyman, 1959: 125–126).

4. Our rationale is consistent with the interpretation by Hyman and Sheatsley (1964: 3) and by Schwartz (1967: 11–12, 28–41) that the increasing acceptance of racial integration between 1942 and 1964 was the outcome of a complex of long-term trends not easily modified by specific, even highly dramatic events like the Supreme Court decision of 1954.

5. The Berkeley "student revolt" took place in 1964–65. Student Health Organizations (SHO's), impatient with the slower-moving and traditionally conservative Student American Medical Association, were organized in 1965, and by 1971 had spread to 70 medical schools. SHO's included medical, nursing, dental, and social work students and emphasized service to the community by multiprofessional teams. Student-run summer community health projects in poverty areas were funded by the Office of Economic Opportunity (McGarvey, Mullan, and Sharfstein, 1968).

6. Foreign Medical Graduate (FMG) housestaff, nearly all of whom were born and reared abroad, and making up about a third of our national housestaff sample, were excluded from this analysis because they constitute different "generations," having been exposed to different historical events and experiences than housestaff raised and trained in the United States. Also, for forecasting the future ideology of the American medical profession, their views should not be considered since about half or more of the FMG housestaff in the mid-seventies planned to return to their home countries (Stevens, Goodman, and Mick, 1978). FMG senior physicians, however, making up about 14 percent of the total, were included in the analysis because they shared more of the American historical experience and the vast majority remained in practice in the United States. Significantly, FMG's were more liberal in their political and government-in-medicine views than USMG's among both senior physicians and housestaff, but the difference was much stronger among the latter (see Colombotos, Kirchner, and Charles, 1977: 605–606).

7. There were puzzling differences, however, between the patterns of the responses of trainees and senior physicians to specific arrangements of practice. Among students and housestaff, the desirability of solo and partnership practice remained quite low and stable according to year in training; and, whereas the "desirability" of a "small group of 3 to 5 physicians in *one* specialty" and of a "large group based in a hospital" increased steadily with year in training, the desirability of a "small, *multi*-specialty group" declined sharply. Among senior physicians, however, the desirability of solo practice increased sharply with age (6% of those under 35 and 34% of those 65 or over considering it desirable), while the desirability of a small, *single*-specialty group practice and of a large, hospital-based group practice dropped.

8. See Campbell et al., 1960: 162; Abramson, 1975: 82; Abramson, 1983. Exceptions to the general pattern in the population are worth noting. For example, the elderly are *more* likely than the young to support governmental involvement in the financing and provision of medical care (Bengtson and Cutler, 1976: 140–143). This pattern, explained in terms of self-interest and group benefits, might conceivably have some bearing in muting the age differences in the views of physicians toward NHI and toward other instances of government participation in health care. But it is hardly relevant to the views of physicians toward other more general and abstract political issues.

9. A longitudinal study of the medical school class of 1979 from the three medical schools in North Carolina between 1975 and 1979 showed that students became more conservative in their political-health care views during this period. Although the author recognized that the changes may be due to "general conservative trends nationally" or to "aging," she argued

that they were more likely the result of the "professional socialization process" (Leserman, 1980: 421). Had the study been done between 1968 and 1972, it would probably have shown, as did the CMA study, that students became more liberal. Would the author have argued that case for "professional socialization" rather than for "general liberal trends nationally"?

10. The processes of "aging," "career stage," and "professional socialization" are of course intertwined empirically, but their effects on attitudes should be distinguished analytically. An attempt to separate the effects of age and career stage (year in training of housestaff and senior physician status) among our housestaff and senior physicians under 35 was disappointing because age and career stage were so closely interrelated. It is worth noting, parenthetically, that although FMG housestaff were much more liberal than U.S. housestaff in their attitudes toward political and government-in-medicine views, they did not differ according to year in training.

11. The comparability of the data is qualified in two ways: (1) The NORC sample is based on a national sample of physicians named by respondents in a population sample as their "regular doctor," thus essentially excluding such specialists as pathologists, radiologists, and anesthesiologists, who, according to our data, are relatively pro-group practice. (2) The questions were worded slightly differently. Our question included the words, "suppose your income in all of these were the same," which probably increased the proportion who chose various types of group practice over individual practice in 1973. The specific group-practice choices were also worded a little differently in the two studies. Although differences between the two periods may be reduced somewhat by these differences in method, their direction is probably not affected.

12. In our study of New York State private practitioners in 1970, older physicians were much more likely than younger ones to favor fixed fees rather than customary fees under Medicare and NHI (Colombotos, 1971: 23).

13. We limit ourselves in this discussion to the findings on the "desirability" of various forms of practice and, by extension, on the perceptions about which of these forms lead to the "best medical care." The curvilinear relationship between career-stage and the "undesirability" of practice arrangements, together with the varied patterns with respect to specific arrangements of practice, described earlier, are too intricate to unravel here.

6 Physicians and Medicare: A Before–After Study of the Effects of Legislation

Seldom has a law been more bitterly opposed by any group than was Medicare by the medical profession (see Feingold, 1966; Harris, 1966; Rose, 1967). Just before Medicare was passed by Congress in 1965, there was even talk about a "boycott" of the program by physicians.[1]

In this chapter, we first examine how physicians responded to Medicare—in thought and in deed—after it was passed and implemented. Next, we examine under what conditions some physicians changed, while others did not change, their attitudes toward Medicare. Then, we look at the extent to which changes in the attitudes of physicians toward Medicare "generalized" to their attitudes toward other political and health care issues. Finally, we compare how physicians responded to Medicare and Medicaid. The underlying question here is: Under what conditions do legislated changes affect attitudes and behavior?

Change in Attitudes Toward Medicare

Law as an Instrument of Social Change

The general issue raised by the question of how physicians responded to Medicare is the role of law as an instrument of social change.

One view, attributed to early sociologists such as Herbert Spencer and William Graham Sumner, is that law can never move ahead of the customs or mores of the people, that legislation which is not rooted in the folkways is doomed to failure. Social change must be slow, and change in public opinion must precede legislative action. In brief, "stateways cannot change folkways."

Others see law as a positive force in initiating social change (Allport,

1954: 471): "It is a well known psychological fact that most people accept the results of an election or legislation gladly enough after the furor has subsided. . . . They allow themselves to be re-educated by the new norm that prevails."

These positions on the role of law as an instrument of social change miss the complexity of the problem. The question must be specified: Under what conditions do laws have what effects?

Effects: Behavior Versus Attitudes

Sumner's negative position on law as an instrument of social change has been distorted, according to one reappraisal of his writings (Ball et al., 1962). In distinguishing between the effects of law on overt behavior and on attitudes, Sumner (1906: 68) did not reject the power of law to influence people's behavior: "Men can always perform the prescribed act, although they cannot always think or feel prescribed thoughts or emotions."

This agrees with the views of most contemporary politically liberal social scientists, who see law primarily as a way of changing behavior, not attitudes. For example: "[Legal action] cannot coerce thoughts or instill subjective tolerance. . . . Law is intended only to control the outward expression of intolerance" (Allport, 1954: 477). And according to MacIver (1954: viii), "No law should require men to change their attitudes. . . . In a democracy we do not punish a man because he is opposed to income taxes, or to free school education, or to vaccination, or to minimum wages, but the laws of a democracy insist that he obey the laws that make provisions for these changes."

The distinction between the effects of law on attitudes and on overt behavior is supported by empirical studies showing a discrepancy between the two (see Deutscher, 1966). In race relations, for example, study after study has shown that in concrete situations—in hotel accommodations (LaPiere, 1934), restaurant service (Kutner et al., 1952), department store shopping (Saenger and Gilbert, 1950), hospital accommodations, and school desegregation (Clark, 1953)—expressions of prejudice are not necessarily accompanied by discriminatory behavior. There are undoubtedly instances of the opposite, that is, verbal expressions of tolerance accompanied by discriminatory behavior, but they are not as well documented. The flight of white, liberal, middle-class families from the cities to the suburbs may be such an instance (Scott and Scott, 1968).

But to say that attitudes and behavior are not perfectly correlated is not to say they are unrelated; there is considerable evidence that change in behavior leads to change in attitudes. Studies of integrated army units, housing projects, and children's camps show that white people in these situations develop more favorable attitudes toward blacks (U.S. War Department, 1945; Deutsch and Collins, 1951; Yarrow, 1958). In an analysis of school desegregation, Hyman and Sheatsley (1964: 6) describe the process thus: "There is obviously some parallel between public opinion and official action. . . . Close analysis of the current findings . . . leads us to the conclusion that in those parts of the South where some measure of school integration has taken place official action has preceded public sentiment, and *public sentiment has then attempted to accommodate itself to the new situation*" (*emphasis added*). (Other studies [e.g., Mussen, 1950; Campbell, 1958], however, have found that social contact has few, or qualified, effects in reducing prejudice.)

If, indeed, behavioral change does lead to attitudinal change, then law, by first changing behavior, may ultimately lead to changes in attitudes. As Allport says; "Outward action, psychology knows, has an eventual effect upon inner habits of thought and feeling. And for this reason we list legislative action as one of the major methods of reducing not only public discrimination [behavior], but private prejudice [attitudes] as well" (1954: 477). Berger, too, writes: "Law does not change attitudes directly, but by altering the situations in which attitudes and opinions are formed, law can indirectly reach the more private areas of life it cannot touch directly in a democratic society" (Berger, 1954: 187). Clark (1953: 72), among others, states the issue in more problematic terms: "Situationally determined changes in behavior [as in response to a law] *may or may not* be accompanied by compatible changes in attitudes or motivation of the individuals involved" (*emphasis added*).

Others, however, see law exerting a *direct* influence on attitudes, without necessarily changing behavior first. Law is conceived as a legitimizing and educational force, supporting one value or set of values against another. For example, according to Dicey (1914: 465): "No facts play a more important part in the creation of opinion than laws themselves." And according to Bonfield (1965: 111): "Past the change in attitude which may be caused by legally mandated and enforced nondiscriminatory conduct, *the mere existence of the law itself affects prejudice*. People usually agree with the law and internalize its values. This is because considerable moral and symbolic weight is added to a principle when it is embedded in legislation" (*emphasis added*).

Others emphasize the fait accompli effect of legislated acts—the perception of their irreversibility. Cantril (1947: 228) notes:

> When an opinion is held by a slight majority or when opinion is not solidly structured, an *accomplished fact* tends to shift opinion in the direction of acceptance. Poll figures show that immediately after the repeal of the arms embargo, immediately after the passage of the conscription laws, and imme-

diately after favorable Congressional action on lend-lease and on the repeal of the neutrality laws [just before the United States' entry into World War II] there was invariably a rise of around ten percent in the number of people favorable to these actions.

Muir (1967) found that the Supreme Court decision banning religious exercise in the nation's schools had an overall positive effect on the attitudes and behavior of officials in one public school system, though there was some evidence of a backlash.

Other studies, however, argue that laws and court decisions have negligible effects on relevant attitudes. Hyman and Sheatsley (1964: 3) and Schwartz (1967: 11-12, 28-41) interpret the increasing acceptance of integration between 1942 and 1964 as a complex of long-term trends that are not easily modified by specific, even highly dramatic events, such as the Supreme Court decision of 1954. The physicians' strike against the province's medical care plan in Saskatchewan, Canada, in 1962 (Badgley and Wolfe, 1967) is an extreme case of noncompliance with a program implemented by a law.[2]

Conditions for Effectiveness of Law

Factors that determine the effectiveness of law include: (1) the degree of compatibility of the law with existing values; (2) the enforceability of the law; (3) the clarity of public policy and the diligence of enforcement.[3]

1. To say that a law must be compatible with some existing values is not to say that it must be compatible with all values. In any society, especially in modern, industrial society, values themselves "are full of inconsistencies and strains, unliberated tendencies in many directions, responsive adjustments to new situations well conceived or ill conceived" (MacIver, 1948: 279). A law, then, "maintains one set of values against another" (Pound, 1944: 25). Thus, desegregation and civil rights laws find support in the democratic creed and due process; Medicare finds support in the principle that adequate medical care is a right, rather than a privilege. This position appears to be in agreement with Sumner's principle of a "strain toward consistency." There is an important difference, however. Whereas Sumner posed the question of compatibility between a new law and existing mores as all or nothing, the current view emphasizes conflicts and strains among a system of mores and poses the question of compatibility as a matter of degree (Myrdal, 1944: 1045-1057).

2. In order for a law to be enforceable, the behavior to be changed must be observable. It is more difficult to enforce a law against homosexual acts, for example, than a law against racial discrimination in public transportation.

3. The authorities responsible must be fully committed to enforcing the new law. One reason for the failure of Prohibition was the failure, or disinclination, of law enforcement agents to implement the law. Civil rights legislation runs into the same problem where local authorities look the other way when aware of discrimination.

We will consider these—and other—conditions below in discussing physicians' reactions to other legislated changes in health care.

The Medicare Law

Medicare, signed into law in July 1965, was a major piece of social legislation. It was often compared in importance with the original Social Security Act of 1935.

Medicare, Title 18 of the Social Security Amendments Act of 1965, established a new program of health insurance for people 65 years old or over. It has two parts; hospital insurance (Part A), applying automatically to almost all people 65 or over, which covers inpatient hospital services, outpatient hospital diagnostic services, and posthospital care in the patient's home or in an extended care facility (such as a nursing home); and medical insurance (Part B), a voluntary plan elected by over 90 percent of those eligible for Part A, which covers physicians' services wherever they are furnished, home health services, and a number of other medical services. Part A is financed by the same method that finances retirement, disability, and death benefits under Social Security, that is, special Social Security contributions by employees and their employers. Part B is financed by a monthly premium from each participant matched from general revenues of the federal government.

For twenty years the American Medical Association fought bitterly and effectively against such a federal program of health insurance under Social Security. But how did individual physicians react, in their behavior and in their attitudes, to Medicare once it became law?

Our data in this part of the analysis come from standardized interviews in 1964 and 1965, before Medicare was passed, with 1,205 physicians in private practice in New York State (about 80% of a probability sample stratified on geographic area and weighted), and from reinterviews with subsamples of these physicians at three different times after Medicare was passed: 1966, 1967, and 1970. In addition, we refer to data from a New York State subsample of 142 office-based practitioners in the 1973 national study.

Among the questions in the first wave of interviews was: "What is your opinion about the bill that would provide for compulsory health insurance through Social Security to cover hospital costs for those over 65—Are you personally in favor of such a plan, or are you opposed to it?"

The bill referred to was passed, as noted above, in July, 1965, as Part A of Title 18. Part B of Title 18, the voluntary insurance plan that pays for physicians' bills and other services, and Title 19 ("Medicaid") which provides for federal matching funds to states for medical care for the "medically indigent," were not covered in the first wave of interviews because they were not introduced in the bill until the Spring of 1965. Title 19, as a matter of fact, received little publicity until after the bill was passed. Thus, before the law was passed, measures were available of physicians' attitudes toward what was generally considered the major feature of the bill, hospital insurance for the elderly, and many related issues, providing a unique opportunity for a natural experiment of the effects of legislation on attitudes.

The 1,205 physicians were stratified on their initial attitude toward Title 18A (i.e., before it was passed) and on geographic area, religious background, and political ideology, all of which were highly correlated with their initial attitude toward Title 18A,[4] and randomly divided into two subsamples, one with 804 and the other with 401 physicians.

The first subsample of 804 physicians was contacted between the middle of May 1966 and the end of June 1966, nearly one year after Medicare was passed and just before it was to go into effect. The second subsample of 401 doctors was contacted between the end of January and April, 1967, a little over six months after the main provisions of the Medicare program had gone into effect. More than 80 percent of each of these subsamples—676 and 331, respectively—were successfully reinterviewed. Of these 1,007 physicians, 828 were successfully reinterviewed a third time in the Spring of 1970, five years after Medicare was passed.

To summarize, 1,205 doctors were interviewed before Medicare was passed (call this Time 1). Of these, 676 were reinterviewed about ten months after the law was passed and just before its implementation (call this Time 2),[5] and another 331 were reinterviewed a little over six months after its implementation (call this Time 3); 828 of these 1,007 were reinterviewed in the spring of 1970 (call this Time 4).[6] The New York State subsample of office-based practitioners in the 1973 national study provides a Time 5 measure on same questions.

Thus, differences in attitudes between Time 1 and Time 2 would reflect the effects of the Medicare law before actual experience with it; differences between Time 1 and Time 3 would reflect the combined effects of the Medicare law and short-term experience with the program; the Time 4 and Time 5 measures would reflect the effects of long-term experience with the program. This design makes it possible to separate the effects on attitudes of the law itself from the effects of its implementation, that is, short-term and long-term experience with the program. The design is presented in Figure 6-1.

Findings

Physicians' Behavior

As the Medicare bill was going through its final stages in Congress in June 1965, resolutions were introduced at the semiannual meeting of the AMA's House of Delegates calling for a "boycott," or "nonparticipation," if it was passed (*New York Times*, June 22, 1965, p. 1). Immediately after the law was passed, the president of the AMA predicted that "quite a few" physicians throughout the country would refuse to participate in the program (*New York Times*, August 18, 1965, p. 55). By the following March, however, it was reported that "threats of boycott, if not dead, are at least moot" (*New York Times*, March 28, 1966, p. 1). When the AMA House of Delegates met in June 1966, a month before Medicare was to go into effect, there was little, if any, talk of a boycott. In fact, there was no boycott, that is, no concerted noncooperation on a large scale.

Responses from the New York State private practitioners interviewed in this study were consistent with the evidence of nationwide compliance by physicians. In the fall of 1965, just a few months after the law was passed, the New York State Medical Society issued a statement that "now that 'Medicare' is an accomplished fact, [the Society] will cooperate in every way possible with the government. . . . As citizens and as physicians, the members of the State Society will obey, and assist in the implementation of the law of the land . . ." (Editorial, *New York State Journal of Medicine*, 1965: 2779).

The physicians interviewed were asked if they agreed or disagreed with their Society's policy of cooperation. Ninety percent agreed at Time 2; 91 percent agreed at Time 3 (see Table 6-1).

At Time 2, less than 5 percent said they would not accept patients who get benefits under Medicare (see Table 6-1). At Time 3, 6 percent of those who had any patients 65 or over had not treated any patients under Title 18B, but only one of the 331 physicians interviewed at that time had actually refused to treat any patients under Title 18B. That doctor explained he was in "semi-retirement" (he was 73 years old, and he wasn't "going to bother with this.") The remainder of the 6 percent indicated that none of their elderly patients had come to them for treatment yet.

To sum up, despite threats of a boycott before Medicare was passed, practically all physicians complied after it became "the law of the land."[7]

Figure 6–1. Research Design of New York State Study

MEDICARE AND MEDICAID BECOME LAW July 30, 1965		*MEDICARE PROGRAM IS IMPLEMENTED* July 1, 1966			
Time 1 January to April, 1964, November, 1964, to March, 1965		*Time 2* May to June, 1966	*Time 3* January to April, 1967	*Time 4* April to July, 1970
Interviews with 1,205 physicians in private practice		Reinterviews with 676 of a stratified subsample of 804 from Time 1. Also, 330 of a control sample of 472 interviewed.	Reinterviews with 331 of remaining stratified subsample of 401 from 1,205 interviewed at Time 1.	Reinterviews with 828 of the 1,007 [676 + 331] physicians interviewed at Time 1 and Time 2 and Time 3. Also, 278 of 330 in Time 2 control sample reinterviewed.

Table 6-1. Responses of Physicians Indicating Compliance with Medicare at Time 2 and Time 3[a]

		Time 2	Time 3
Last fall the New York State Medical Society said it would co-operate with the government on Medicare—do you agree or disagree with this policy?[b]			
	Agree	90%	91%
	Disagree	8	8
	Don't know, no answer	2	1
		100%	100%
	Base N's	(676)	(331)
According to your present thinking, do you plan to accept patients who get benefits-under Medicare, or not?[c]			
	Accept (have treated)	93%	93%
	Will not accept (have not treated)	4	6
	Don't know, no answer	4	1
		101%	100%
	Base N's	(609)	(299)

[a]"Time 1" in these tables refers to interviews conducted before the passage of Medicare, from January to April, 1964, and from November, 1964, to March, 1965; "Time 2," to interviews done after the passage of Medicare but before its implementation, from May to June, 1966; "Time 3," to interviews done after the implementation of Medicare, from January to April, 1967.

[b]This is the Time 2 question. The Time 3 question was: "The New York State Medical Society has said it would cooperate with the government on both Titles 18 and 19. Regarding Title 18, do you agree or disagree with this policy?"

[c]This is the Time 2 question. The Time 3 question was: "Have you treated any patients who get benefits under Part B of Title 18, or not?" The figures for both questions exclude those physicians who indicated in a previous question that they had no patients 65 years of age or over.

Of the 18 physicians with patients 65 or over who had not treated any of these patients under Title 18B at Time 3, only one had actually refused. The others reported that no elderly patients had come to them for treatment since Medicare.

Physicians' Attitudes

It is possible, of course, for physicians to comply with Medicare without changing their minds about it. What effects did Medicare have on physicians' attitudes toward the program? In 1964 and early 1965, before Medicare was passed (Time 1), 38 percent of the private practitioners in New York State were "in favor" of "the bill that would provide for compulsory health insurance through Social Security to cover hospital costs for those over 65," the bill that became Title 18A. This was a sizeable number, but nevertheless, a minority.

At Time 2, ten months after the law was passed, even before it went into effect, the proportion "in favor" jumped to 70 percent. At Time 3, only six months after the program went into effect, the proportion "in favor" again jumped, to 81 percent. At both Time 2 and Time 3, more than half of those in favor felt "strongly," rather than only "somewhat" in favor (see Table 6-2). At Time 4, 92 percent favored Medicare, 63 percent "strongly," and only 6 percent opposed it. (It remained at this level in 1973, when 91 percent of the New York State office-based practitioners in the national study sample were in favor of Medicare.)

Table 6-3 shows that of those opposed to Title 18A at Time 1, more than half (59%) had switched by Time 2; 70 percent had switched by Time 3.[8] Very few switched from favoring it to opposing it.

Although the absolute percentage increase favoring Title 18A of Medicare was greater between Time 1 and Time 2 (from 38 to 70%), than between Time 2 and Time 3 (from 70 to 81%) and between Time 3 and Time 4 (from 81 to 92%), it might be misleading, because of the operation of a "ceiling effect," to argue that the Medicare law itself had a stronger impact than experience of the physicians with the program implemented by the law.[9] What can be asserted, however, is that the law itself had a large effect on physicians' attitudes toward Medicare even before it was implemented.

Table 6-2. Attitudes of Physicians Toward Medicare (Title 18A) at Time 1, Time 2, Time 3, and Time 4[a]

	Time 1	Time 2	Time 3	Time 4
Favor	38%	70%	81%	92%
Strongly		38	45	63
Somewhat		31	33	28
Don't know, no answer		1	3	1
Oppose	54	26	19	6
Strongly		14	10	3
Somewhat		11	9	3
Don't know, no answer		1	*	—
Don't know, no answer	8	5	*	2
	100%	101%	100%	100%
Base N's	(1,205)	(676)	(331)	(828)

[a]At Time 1, the question was: "What is your opinion about the bill that would provide for compulsory health insurance through Social Security to cover hospital costs for those over 65—are you personally in favor of such a plan, or are you opposed to it?" Respondents were not asked whether they were "strongly" or "somewhat" in favor or opposed at Time 1.

At Time 2 and Time 4 the questions were: "What is your opinion of Part A of Medicare—the part that provides for compulsory health insurance through Social Security to cover hospital costs for those over 65—are you personally in favor of this plan, or opposed to it?" "Would you say strongly (in favor) (opposed) or somewhat (in favor) (opposed)?" At Time 3 the words "Part A of Title 18" were substituted for the words "Part A of Medicare."

*Less than 0.5 percent.

Table 6-3. Attitudes of Physicians Toward Medicare (Title 18A) at Time 2 and Time 3 by Their Attitudes at Time 1

	Time 1 attitude toward Medicare	
	Favor	Oppose
Time 2 attitude toward Medicare		
Favor	90%	59%
Strongly	59	25
Somewhat	30	33
Don't know, no answer	1	1
Oppose	11	40
Strongly	5	22
Somewhat	6	16
Don't know, no answer	0	2
	101%	99%
Base N's	(256)	(348)
Time 3 attitude toward Medicare		
Favor	98%	70%
Strongly	84	19
Somewhat	10	48
Don't know, no answer	4	3
Oppose	2	30
Strongly	*	17
Somewhat	2	13
Don't know, no answer	0	*
	100%	100%
Base N's	(123)	(185)

*Less than 0.5 percent.

Consistent with the increase in the level of physicians' support for Medicare between Time 2 and Time 3 is the fact that they were less worried about the consequences of Medicare at Time 3 than at Time 2 (unfortunately, our Time 1 interview did not include questions about these perceived consequences); their earlier fears simply did not material- ize.[10] For example, the proportion who thought that the quality of care physicians give their elderly patients would be "not as good" under Medicare dropped from 28 percent at Time 2 to 8 percent at Time 3 (see Table 6-4). The proportion who thought there would be "a great deal" or "a fair amount" of unnecessary hospitalization under Medicare dropped from 69 percent at Time 2 to 38 percent at Time 3 (27% thought there had actually been "a great deal" or "a fair amount" of unnecessary hospitalization up to Time 3). The proportion who thought there would be "a great deal" or "a fair amount" of unnecessary utilization of physicians' services under Medicare also dropped from 77 percent to 36 percent (25% thought there had actually been "a great deal" or "a fair amount" up to Time 3). It is only in the questions about government interference under Medicare and its effects on physicians' income that there were not significant changes, but only 12 percent at Time 2 and 11 percent at Time 3 thought that they would earn less money under Medicare than before, compared with more than a third who thought they would earn more money.[11]

At Time 4, when physicians were asked to what extent they perceived that these concerns had in fact materialized, we find a mixed picture. They were a little more likely to perceive unnecessary utilization of the services of both hospitals and physicians than they had expected at Time 3. On the other hand, they were more likely to think that doctors earned more money under Medicare and that the federal government had in fact interfered with the individual doctor's professional freedom "very little" or "not at all."

Alternative Interpretations

Let us consider some alternative explanations of the large shifts in attitude toward Medicare:

1. It could be argued that the changes described above could have taken place without the Medicare law and its implementation; that the shift in physicians' attitudes toward Medicare was part of a general, long-term liberal trend in their thinking. Obviously, there was not available a control group of physicians from whom the facts of the passage of the Medicare law and its implementation could be withheld. The argument that the changes in attitude toward Medicare were due to the actual adoption of the law, however, is supported by the following observations:

a. The change in attitude toward Title 18A was a large change from 38 percent in favor to 70 to 81 percent within a period of three years. It is not plausible to argue that this was due to a general ideological trend unrelated to the passage and implementation of Medicare.

b. The attitudes that did change were highly specific to Medicare. Physicians' responses to questions indicating their position on economic-welfare issues, political party preference, group practice, and peer reviews, all of which were strongly related to their attitudes toward Title 18A at Time 1, were relatively stable compared with their responses

Table 6-4. Perceived Effects of Medicare (Title 18) at Time 2 and at Time 3

	Time 2	Time 3	Time 4[a]
Base N's	(676)	(331)	(828)
In your opinion, how will Medicare (Title 18) affect the *quality* of care doctors give their elderly patients—in general, will doctors give *better* medical care, or *not as good* care, or won't Medicare (Title 18) make any difference?			
Better	14	30	36
Not as good	28	8	6
No difference	54	60	52
Don't know	5	2	6
	100%	100%	100%
In your opinion, will there be a great deal of *unnecessary hospitalization* under Medicare (Title 18), or a fair amount, or very little, or none at all?			
Great deal	32	12	16
Fair amount	37	26	34
Very little	18	38	29
None at all	9	20	11
Don't know	4	4	9
	100%	100%	100%
Will there be a great deal of *unnecessary* utilization of *doctors' services* under Medicare (Title 18), or a fair amount, or very little, or none at all?			
Great deal	39	8	13
Fair amount	38	28	35
Very little	15	39	31
None at all	4	20	13
Don't know	4	5	8
	100%	100%	100%

to the question on Medicare. If the change in attitudes toward Medicare were part of a more general trend in physicians' thinking and unrelated to the passage of Medicare, then one would expect changes in attitudes toward these other issues as well.

2. It could be argued that the increasingly favorable medical opinion about Medicare and the passage of the Medicare law were both the result or part of a third factor occurring immediately before Medicare was passed. Strong public support for Medicare, for example, could have influenced both medical and legislative opinion. Data in the present study from two independent samples of Manhattan doctors who were interviewed at two different times before Medicare was passed do not

Table 6-4. Perceived Effects of Medicare (Title 18) at Time 2 and at Time 3 (*Continued*)

	Time 2	Time 3	Time 4[a]
Base N's	(676)	(331)	(828)

In your opinion, will doctors *earn more* money under Medicare (Title 18) than before, or less money, or won't Medicare (Title 18) make any difference?

	Time 2	Time 3	Time 4
More	35	42	59
Less	12	11	2
No difference	41	38	29
Don't know	12	9	10
	100%	100%	100%

In your opinion, will the Federal government, under Medicare (Title 18), interfere with the individual doctor's professional freedom—Would you say a great deal, or a fair amount, or very little, or not at all?

	Time 2	Time 3	Time 4
Great deal	17	21	6
Fair amount	37	26	16
Very little	25	31	40
Not at all	15	16	36
Don't know	6	6	3
	100%	100%	100%

[a] At Time 4, physicians were asked to what extent they perceived that given consequences were materializing or had materialized. They were asked "How has Medicare affected the care doctors give their elderly patients. . . ?"; "Has there been so far a great deal of unnecessary hospitalization. . . ?"; and so on.

support such an argument. The first sample of 70 physicians was interviewed from January to April in 1964, about 18 months before Medicare was passed. The second sample of 61 physicians was interviewed from November, 1964, to March, 1965, barely six months before the law was passed. There was essentially no difference in the proportion in favor of Title 18A in the two samples—53 percent in the first sample, 57 percent in the second.

3. It is possible that the acceptance of Medicare by New York State physicians after the enactment of the law was influenced by their opposition to the state's Medicaid program. The implementation of Medicaid in New York State was one of the most liberal in the country. The first version of the New York State program was signed into law on April 30, 1966. The program was amended and curtailed two months later after strong opposition in upstate New York and threatened boycotts by county medical societies.

At Time 2, just after the first version of Medicaid was passed by the state legislature, 42 percent of the doctors interviewed said they were in favor of the law. At Time 3, despite, or perhaps because of, the fact the program had been curtailed six months earlier, it was still only 42 percent; at Time 4, only 45 percent favored Medicaid.

On all other questions about Medicaid asked at Time 3, it was less well received than Medicare:

a. Forty-six percent thought that the government would interfere "a great deal" with the professional freedom of individual physicians under Medicaid, compared with 21 percent for Medicare.

b. Fifty-nine percent thought that the state medical society should cooperate with the government on Medicaid, compared with 91 percent on Medicare.

c. Fifty-five percent said they planned to accept (or had already accepted) patients under Title 19, compared with all but one physician under Title 18B.

It could be argued that the opposition to Medicaid in New York State had a "contrast" effect on the responses of physicians to Medicare; that Medicare looked better to physicians than it would have looked had Medicaid not been passed, and that this "contrast" inflated the size of the oppose–favor switchers on Medicare. For example, at the height of the furor over Medicaid in the state, one county medical society in an advertisement in *The New York Times* agreed to "cooperate" with the "Federal Medicare Law, which provides a sensible and reasonable plan of medical care for all people over 65," but found it "impossible to cooperate with the implementation of this State law [Medicaid] . . . as it is presently proposed" (June 10, 1966, p. 36). It called Medicaid "socialized medicine."

There is no evidence of such a contrast effect in our data. Rather, among those physicians who opposed Title 18A at Time 2, those who were in *favor* of Medicaid at Time 2 and Time 3 were much more likely than those who opposed Medicaid to switch and favor Title 18A.[12]

4. It could be argued that the physicians' attitudes toward Medicare expressed before its passage were superficial and equivocal, and merely reflected official AMA policy; and that once the program became law, physicians felt freer to express their "real" attitudes toward Medicare. But this argument is simply another way of making the point that law may "legitimate" opinion. The fact that the Medicare program was not law is as significant a part of the social situation in the expression of physicians' attitudes as the fact that it later became law. Conversely, one could just as plausibly argue for the "superficiality" of attitudes expressed after the law was on the books, because of a "bandwagon effect," as for the "superficiality" of attitudes expressed before the law was passed.

As a matter of fact, neither at Time 1 nor at Time 2 and Time 3 did the

attitudes toward Medicare appear superficial. The subquestion on intensity of feeling was not asked at Time 1. In the Time 1 measure, however,
fewer than 8 percent responded "don't know." Also, attitudes toward
Medicare at Time 1 were strongly related to other political questions and
issues in the organization of medical practice (Colombotos, 1968), which
argues against its superficiality. In the Time 2 and 3 measures, the
number of "don't knows" was even smaller than at Time 1: at Time 2, it
was 5 percent, and at Time 3, it was less than 0.5 percent. Also, of those
in favor, more than half responded they felt "strongly" in favor, rather
than only "somewhat" in favor.[13]

Since none of these alternative explanations of the large shift in attitude toward Medicare is supported, our argument that the change is a real
one and attributable to the passage and implementation of the law is
thereby strengthened.

In summary, despite their opposition to Medicare before the law was
passed in 1965, physicians complied with the program. Consistent with
their compliance, a large number of physicians who were opposed to
Medicare before it became law switched and accepted it after it became
law.[14] The large increase in the proportion favoring Medicare between
Time 1 (before the law) and Time 2 (after its adoption, but before its
implementation) supports the argument that for law to influence attitudes it does not *necessarily* have to change relevant behavior first. We
have in the response of physicians to Medicare a case in which attitudes
adapted to the law even before it went into effect.

These results support the interpretation that legislation had a legitimizing and fait accompli effect. But changes in physicians' *perceptions* of
the substantive impact of Medicare may have also contributed to its
acceptance. We reported earlier that the fears of physicians of the possible
negative effects of Medicare on the quality of care, utilization, their
professional freedom, and their income declined over time. Earlier fears
proved ill-founded. The medical profession was still in control; physicians' income was not about to suffer. As a matter of fact, Medicare
initially supported the stability of physicians' income, without controlling their fees. As Somers and Somers (1967: 1) put it soon after Medicare
was passed:

> The 1965 enactment of Medicare was heralded as "revolutionary." But, in
> fact, it was neither a sudden nor radical departure from the march of events
> in the organization and financing of medical care and government's grow-
> ing participation. No existing institutions were overturned or seriously
> threatened by the new legislation. On the contrary, Medicare responded to
> the needs of the providers of care as well as those of the consumers. It was
> primarily a financial underpinning of the existing health care industry—
> with all that implies in terms of strengths and weaknesses.

But not all physicians switched in support of Medicare. Even at Time 4, five years after its passage, nearly 10 percent continued to oppose it. Among the conditions for the effectiveness of law reviewed earlier were the degree of compatibility of the law with existing values. In that discussion, the units of analysis were individual laws and the social situations into which they were introduced. Here we examine the perceptions and attitudes of individuals as conditions under which they changed their attitudes toward Medicare.

Were the consequences that physicians perceived and expected earlier concerning Medicare—and their prior attitudes toward related issues—related, in turn, to whether or not they switched? Were younger physicians more likely to change than older physicians, thus suggesting an interaction between this "period" effect and age—a question raised in the last chapter? We turn briefly to these questions next.[15]

Conditions of Individual Attitude Change

Perceived Effects of Medicare

We predicted that among physicians opposed to Medicare at a given time, those who expected Medicare to have negative effects would be less likely than those who expected Medicare to have positive effects to switch and favor Medicare at a subsequent time; and that among those in favor of Medicare at a given time, those who expected negative effects would be more likely than those who expected positive effects to switch and oppose Medicare at a subsequent time. Our reasoning is based on the assumption that there is a tendency for perceptions and attitudes to be consistent, as discussed in Chapter 2.

As we indicated earlier, our Time 1 interview did not include questions on physicians' expectations of the effects of Medicare. Physicians' expectations at Time 2 and Time 3 of the effects of Medicare on the quality of care and on their professional freedom were related, as predicted, to changes in their attitudes toward Medicare by Time 4; but their expectations of the effects on physicians' income and on overutilization were not related to such changes.[16]

Attitudes Toward Related Political and Health Care Issues

We predicted that among physicians who opposed Medicare before its passage, those with liberal political views and those who supported group practice and peer reviews were more likely to change their attitudes toward Medicare than those with conservative political views and those who opposed group practice and peer reviews. These attitudes were intercorrelated among private practitioners in New York State before Medicare (Colombotos, 1968), just as they were intercorrelated among the national sample in 1973, as discussed in Chapter 2. The reasoning under-lying our predictions appeals, again, to the concept of consistency.

As an example, consider a Democrat opposed to Medicare before its passage (Time 1)—an inconsistent pattern. He could become consistent by supporting Medicare, or by becoming a Republican. The legitimation of Medicare by its passage into law (plus the more general and more longstanding character of party preference) would make a change in attitude toward Medicare the more likely way of resolving the conflict than a change in party preference. A Democrat in favor of Medicare at Time 1 represents a consistent, and therefore presumably stable, pattern. The stability of this pattern is further strengthened by Medicare's becom-ing law.

Now, consider Republican physicians. Those who opposed Medicare at Time 1 were consistent. Despite this being a consistent and stable pattern, however, we would expect some Republican opponents of Medi-care to change and support Medicare once it became law. The proportion of initial opponents of Medicare among Republicans who change, how-ever, should be lower than among the Democrats, for whom opposition to Medicare was an inconsistent position.

Although favoring Medicare before it was passed was an inconsistent position for Republicans, we would expect some of them to maintain this inconsistent position because of the legitimizing effect of the law; but we would expect a higher proportion of Time 1 supporters of Medicare to defect among the Republicans (inconsistents) than among the Democrats (consistents).

Our findings indicate that physicians' views toward political and gov-ernment-in-health issues generally did influence whether they changed their attitudes toward Medicare, and in the direction predicted. Their attitudes toward health care issues did not have such an effect, however, perhaps because they were not as strongly related to their attitudes toward Medicare, to begin with.[17]

Age

In the last chapter we raised the possibility that older people may be more resistant than younger people to the effects of new events. Among physi-cians opposed to Medicare at a given time, were the older less likely than the younger to change their minds and subsequently support it? Our data show they were not. In fact, there was a slight tendency for the older to be more likely than the younger to switch between Time 1 and Times 2, 3.

Generalization of Changes in Attitudes: Medicare and Other Issues

What were the *effects* of the changes in physicians' attitudes toward Medicare on their attitudes toward other issues—on their political views and on their attitudes toward health care issues, all of which were correlated with their attitude toward Medicare before the law was passed? Did the acceptance of Medicare by physicians make them more liberal and more receptive to other changes in the health care system? Or did opposition to further change stiffen?

We have already reported that there was little short-term effect, that is, right after Medicare was passed, on these issues. The stability of these attitudes over the short run was offered, as a matter of fact, to support the argument that the change in attitudes toward Medicare was indeed an effect of the Medicare law rather than a part of a more general liberal trend in the thinking of physicians.

Katz (1960: 199) has noted that "it is puzzling that attitude change seems to have slight generalization effects, when the evidence indicates considerable generalization in the organization of a person's beliefs and values." For example, in the field of race relations, there is little evidence that changes in attitudes toward desegregation in a work situation rub off on changes in attitudes toward other forms of desegregation, such as housing and education.

But our results at Time 2 and Time 3, and Katz's observation, refer to the short run. It is plausible to expect that a change in one part of an attitude structure will produce changes in other parts of that structure, but not necessarily immediately. It may take some time for these secondary changes to take place. (One might refer to this as a "domino theory" of attitude change.) It is therefore not surprising that there is little evidence of generalization in research on attitude change, since few such studies extend over a period of more than a year or two. The main purpose of our Time 4 measure—five years after Medicare was passed— was to test the effects of generalization over a longer period of time. The incorporation of the New York State private practitioners in the 1973 national study gives us a still later measure on some questions.

The effects were quite differentiated. The attitudes of physicians toward the organizational issues of health care (group practice, peer reviews, and task delegation) on the one hand, and toward *general* political issues (economic-welfare issues, political identification, and political party preference) on the other, were quite stable over the period. There were strong trends, however, on issues that were logically (or psychologically) closer to Medicare. There was a consistent increase in the proportion of practitioners who accepted the role of the government in health care. The proportion agreeing with the principle of health care as a right ("it is the responsibility of the [entire] society, through its government, to provide everyone with the best available medical care, whether he can afford it or not") rose steadily, but slowly at first, from 60 percent in 1964, to 80 percent in 1973. One-fifth believed that Medicare did not "go far enough in providing medical care" to the elderly at Time 2 and Time 3, 40 percent, at Time 4, and 45 percent, at "Time 5" (1973)—a steady increase. (The question was not asked at Time 1.)

As measured by other questions, the perceptions of physicians concerning the adequacy of government-sponsored medical care were, however, more volatile. The proportion who thought that "not enough is being done in this country to provide medical care for people who don't have much money," that the federal government "should do more in the field of health," and that there was a "need for more legislation for medical care for the aged," dropped sharply after the passage of Medicare (at Time 2 and Time 3), but rose again by Time 4, on the first two questions to a point higher than that at Time 1. (Apparently, a sizeable number of physicians who thought that Medicare would go a long way toward meeting the country's health needs realized, once the program had been in effect for a while, that it did not go as far as they had hoped—or feared.) As we observed earlier in this chapter, physicians were generally less likely to perceive negative effects of Medicare as time went on.

These were significant trends, for they suggest an increasing acceptance by physicians of the general principle of governmental responsibility in the provision of health care following the passage of Medicare.[18]

Under What Conditions Do Laws Affect Attitudes and Behavior? The Case of Medicare and Medicaid

We contrasted earlier in this chapter the ready accommodation of physicians to Medicare with their continuing opposition to Medicaid. What accounts for these differences? Here we move from individual physicians and subgroups of physicians back to laws as units of analysis. The general question is, under what conditions do laws influence attitudes and behavior?

Differences between Medicare and the New York State Medicaid law illustrate some of the conditions listed above and suggest others that promote the effectiveness of a law:

1. *Medicare and Medicaid differed sharply ideologically and philo-sophically.* Medicare was based on the insurance principle, closely linked with Social Security; Medicaid was based on the welfare principle. The clients of Medicare were the elderly; the clients of Medicaid were the "medically indigent" and identified with "welfare" cases.

New York State's Medicaid affected the practices of physicians much more directly than Medicare. Medicaid attempted to control the quality and cost of medical care: the quality, by establishing criteria for determining who could render care, thus limiting the free choice of physicians; and the cost, by paying physicians fixed fees rather than "usual and customary" charges. Medicare attempted neither, until recently. The direct effects of Medicare on the practices of physicians, as we noted earlier, were quite minimal. Rather, Medicare supported the stability of physicians' income without controlling their fees.

Both in terms of consistency with their ideology and in terms of their self-interest, then, Medicare was more acceptable to New York State physicians than Medicaid.

2. *Degree of popular support.* Medicare was passed with overwhelming popular support. Two-thirds of the public were in favor of Medicare, according to a nationwide Gallup poll in January, 1965, six months before it was passed. The percentage was probably higher in New York State. In contrast, there was little awareness about Medicaid before it was passed, and there was strong opposition, particularly in upstate New York, from industry, farm organizations, and in the press, after the first version of the New York Medicaid law was passed in April, 1966.

3. *Medicare was the same throughout the country, whereas Medicaid varied greatly from state to state.* It is possible that the opposition of New York physicians to their state's Medicaid program, the most liberal in the country, was reinforced by their feeling "worse off" than their colleagues in other states, where the Medicaid programs were not as ambitious (an instance of "relative deprivation"). A plausible hypothesis, setting aside regional and local differences in values that may or may not be congruent with a given law, is that a national law is more "legitimate" and more likely to be effectively complied with than a state or local law.[19]

Summary

The sharp change in the attitudes of physicians toward Medicare following its passage, and even before physicians had any experience with the program, is testimony to the legitimizing and fait accompli effects of legislation. Central to the idea of fait accompli is the perception of its irreversibility. The sense of "accomplished fact" before an event takes place, an "anticipatory" fait accompli, is captured by perceptions of its inevitability. (Some would call it "fatalism.") We reported in Chapter 2 that more than 80 percent of physicians in the early seventies thought that NHI was inevitable, most within five years, and that the attitudes of individual physicians toward NHI were strongly related to their perceptions of its inevitability and imminence. Physicians' support for NHI dropped in the late seventies, because, it is plausible to argue, NHI was no longer viewed as inevitable. But firmer support for the effects of the anticipatory fait accompli effect would be gained by tracking changes over time in physicians' perceptions of the inevitability of, say, NHI, linked to external events, such as the introduction of NHI bills in Congress, changes in political and public support, media content, and the like, and relating changing perceptions to changing attitudes. A resurrection of NHI would provide an opportunity for such a test.

Changes in the attitudes of physicians toward Medicare did indeed rub off on their attitudes toward some other issues (e.g., the role of government in health care), but not on their attitudes toward others. The precise timing of these secondary changes and why some attitudes in a structure are affected by an initial change while others are not remain interesting questions to pursue. It makes sense to assume that the "closer" the content of two attitudes in a structure and the stronger their initial statistical association, the more likely one attitude is to change following a change in the other. But to identify the dimensions defining "closeness" between two or more attitudes is not a simple matter. The identification of changes in the *structure* of attitudes, for example, whether the attitudes of physicians toward health care issues have become more politicized since Medicare, also merits study.

The accommodation of physicians to Medicare, but not to Medicaid, raises the question: under what conditions do legislated changes affect the attitudes and behavior of physicians? Medicare and Medicaid differed sharply with respect to their content, the degree of popular support, and their uniformity throughout the nation. Certainly this line of analysis would be enriched by considering other case studies of how physicians respond to health programs. In the concluding chapter we discuss how physicians are likely to respond to NHI in the next decade, taking into account the findings discussed in the present chapter. Additionally, to what extent are the responses of physicians to one piece of legislation, such as NHI, influenced by their prior experience with another, such as Medicare? Will their relatively easy acceptance of Medicare and their subsequent favorable experiences with it make acceptance of NHI easier than it would have been without the precedent of Medicare?

Notes

1. The AMA's opposition to Medicare before its passage apparently was supported by the majority of its membership. In a national poll of private practitioners in 1961 less than 20 percent were in favor of the program "to provide hospital and nursing home care for the aged through the Social Security System" (*Medical Tribune*, May 15, 1961).

2. In an experimental study, information that a behavior was illegal did not change the subjects' attitudes toward that behavior (Walker and Argyle, 1964). In a followup experiment, however, it was found that knowledge of the law and knowledge of peer consensus did change attitudes, and, furthermore, these effects depended on the authoritarianism of the subjects (Berkowitz and Walker, 1967).

3. These conditions were discussed in: Clark, 1953: 53–59; Berger, 1954: 173–177; Allport, 1954: 469–473; Roche and Gordon, 1960; Rose, 1959; Bonfield, 1965; Evan, 1965; Mayhew, 1968: 258–284. Problems of implementation, specifically, the work and effects of antidiscrimination enforcement agencies, are analyzed by Berger (1954) and Mayhew (1968).

Less commonly cited factors determining the effectiveness of law are: (1) the degree and intensity of opposition. The larger the amount of opposition to the law and the more concentrated the opposition is in politically relevant units, along geographical or occupational lines, for example, then the more effective is the opposition to the law (Roche and Gordon, 1960). (2) The quality of support. A law is more likely to be effective if supported than if it is opposed by community leaders (see Killian, 1958). (3) The tempo of change. It is argued that the less the transition time, the easier the adaptation to the change enacted by the law (see Clark, 1953: 43–47; Evan, 1965: 290, Badgley and Wolfe, 1967: 45).

4. Physicians in New York City were more pro-Medicare than physicians in upstate New York: Jewish physicians were more pro-Medicare than Protestant physicians, with Catholics in between; and those who were Democrats and took a liberal position on economic-welfare issues were more pro-Medicare than were those who were Republicans and took a conservative position (see Colombotos, 1968: 320–331).

5. The 676 physicians interviewed at Time 2 included 100 who could not be reached by June 30 and were interviewed between July and October, after Medicare went into effect. Those interviewed after June 30 were a little better informed than those interviewed before June 30 about the services covered by the Medicare program, which is not surprising, but the patterns of change in the attitude toward Title 18A of the two groups were practically the same. The specific month within the Time 2 or Time 3 periods when respondents were interviewed also made no difference in the pattern of change in their attitude toward Title 18A.

6. The original plan of this phase of the study was to reinterview all 1,205 physicians just before Medicare went into effect and again three to four years after it had been in effect. It was decided, however, to set aside a third of this sample (401) to be reinterviewed six months after the law was implemented in order to test the *short-run* effects of implementation. The original sample of 1,205 was not reinterviewed both before and immediately after Medicare's implementation because of the financial cost and because of a concern about a high refusal rate in the third interview, since the two interviews would come so closely together.

7. Our measures of compliance, apart from being reports of their own behavior rather than observations of their actual behavior, were admittedly simple measures of a complex variable. Consider the following: (1) A physician could provide some services under Medicare, but refuse to provide other services; (2) he or she could provide services to some patients, but refuse to provide them to other patients; (3) he or she could cooperate at one

point in time after the program went into effect, and not cooperate at another; (4) he or she could sabotage the program by "overcomplying," that is, by providing more services than are medically indicated. Also, the question of compliance was irrelevant for physicians without patients 65 or over, such as pediatricians.

As a matter of fact, when the specific behaviors required of physicians under Medicare are examined, it is difficult to conceive what form a boycott of Medicare by physicians could have taken. What was a physician asked to do under Medicare?

(1) A physician had to certify that the diagnostic or therapeutic services for which payment was claimed are "medically necessary." Such certification could be entered on a form or order or prescription the physician ordinarily signed.

(2) Under Title 18, Part B, a physician could choose between two methods of payment for his or her services: accept an assignment and bill a designated carrier (such as Blue Shield, or another private insurance company, depending on the geographic area), or bill the patient directly. If a physician took an assignment, he or she agreed that the "reasonable charge" determined by the carrier would be the full charge and that the physician's charge to the patient would be no more than 20 percent of that reasonable charge. If the physician refused to take an assignment and billed the patient directly, the patient paid the physician, and then applied to the carrier for payment. Under this method, a physician was not restricted by the "reasonable charge" for a given service. The patient, however, was reimbursed only 80 percent of the reasonable charge by the carrier. Although the Social Security Administration had hoped for wide use of the assignment method, the AMA's House of Delegates adopted a resolution at its 1966 meeting recommending the use of the direct billing method (*New York Times*, June 30, 1966, p. 1). Use of the direct billing method could not be called "noncooperation," however, since the law provided for either method.

(3) In order to promote the most efficient use of facilities, each participating hospital and extended care facility was required to have a utilization review plan. A committee set up for such a purpose must include at least two physicians. Many hospitals already had such review procedures before Medicare went into effect. One way in which a physician could protest against Medicare was to refuse to serve on such a committee if asked. But refusal to serve did not necessarily mean a protest against Medicare, any more than unwillingness to run for a local Board of Education is necessarily an indication of protest against the public school system.

In sum, the direct and immediate effects of Medicare on a physician's day-to-day practice were minimal. For the vast majority of services under Medicare, the physician was not required to do anything more or differently in treating patients than before Medicare was passed. One form a boycott of Medicare could have taken would have been for physicians to refuse to treat patients 65 or over, most of whom are eligible for benefits under both Part A and Part B of Medicare. This, apparently, few physicians chose to do. Furthermore, it would be difficult to interpret such acts as "noncooperation," unless the physician said so. In any given case, a physician's refusal to admit an elderly patient to the hospital, for example, could mean that, in his or her medical judgment, hospitalization was not necessary.

8. The attitudes of physicians toward Title 18B were highly correlated with their attitudes toward Title 18A. Seventy-eight percent were "in favor" at Time 2 and 83 percent at Time 3.

9. The effect of an experimental variable on a group is limited by the initial frequency giving a certain response before exposure to that variable. Since the percentage in favor of Medicare is higher at Time 2 than at Time 1, there is "less room" for an increase in the percentage in favor between Time 2 and Time 3 than between Time 1 and Time 2. The

statistical effect of this "ceiling" may be "corrected" by dividing the actual percentage difference by the maximum possible increase. Hovland et al. (1949: 285–289) call such a measure the "effectiveness index." Such an index for the Time 1-Time 2 change is .52 (70−38)/(100−38)=.52. For the Time 2-Time 3 change it is .37 (81−70)/(100−70)=.37. For the Time 3-Time 4 change it is .48 (92−81)/(100−81)=.58. The fact that the Time 1-Time 2 index is larger than the Time 2-Time 3 measure indicates that the larger increase in the percentage of those in favor of Medicare between Time 1 and Time 2 than between Time 2 and Time 3 cannot be explained away as being entirely due to a statistical ceiling effect.

There is another type of "ceiling" effect, this one due to *selection.* Those still opposed to Medicare at Time 2 are likely to include a higher proportion of "hardcore" opponents of Medicare were no more conservative on other measures of political ideology at Time 1 than the Time 1 opponents.

Finally, since we have only one measure of the attitudes of physicians after the law was passed and before its implementation, it is not possible to assess the effect of time alone. It is possible that the change in attitude toward Medicare between Time 2 and Time 3 was a function of time and had nothing to do with the implementation of the program.

10. Clark (1953: 47-50) reports a similar pattern in cases of desegregation.

11. There was no increase in the level of physicians' knowledge about the details of Medicare between Time 2 and 3—they were poorly informed at both times—and there was no association between their level of knowledge and the amount of experience with Medicare, on the one hand, and change in their attitude toward Medicare, on the other.

12. Another test of the effects of Medicaid on attitude change toward Title 18A would be to examine the problem in a state where physicians' attitudes toward Title 18A were similar to those in New York State, but where the Medicaid Program did not arouse as much opposition as the one in New York State. Unfortunately, such data were not available.

13. A number of methodological problems in panel surveys could also have been involved, but were not:

(1) *Reinterview effect.* It could be argued that the Time 1 interview generated an interest in Medicare, thus influencing the responses of physicians in the Time 2 interview. We found no difference between the responses to selected questions, including the one on Medicare, obtained from the reinterviewed sample at Time 2 and from a control sample of 330 physicians not interviewed at Time 1.

(2) *Change in the interview instrument,* specifically in the sequence of the questions. The items preceding the question on Medicare in the Time 2 interview were different from those in the Time 1 interview. We found no difference between the responses obtained in two different versions of the interview at Time 2: one in which the repeat (retest) questions were mixed with new questions and one in which the repeat (retest) questions were asked first, followed by the new questions.

(3) *Mortality effect.* It could be argued that physicians in the panel not interviewed at Time 2 and Time 3 were less likely to be pro-Medicare than those who were interviewed. We found that physicians who could not be reinterviewed at Time 2 and Time 3 did not differ from those who were reinterviewed in either background characteristics or attitudes, including their attitude toward Medicare, expressed at Time 1.

14. New York State physicians are more likely than those in the rest of the country to have liberal political views and to be pro-Medicare. As indicated earlier (Note 1), less than a fifth of a national sample were in favor of Medicare before the law; in 1973, 82 percent of our total national sample were in favor, compared with 93 percent of all New York State physicians.

15. We also examined the effects of social context on physicians (e.g., the level of physician support for Medicare in a geographic area) and of their perceptions of their colleagues' attitudes toward Medicare at a given point in time as conditions for consequent change in their attitudes toward Medicare, but the results of this analysis were negative.

16. In Chapter 2 we observed that physicians' expectations of the effects of NHI on doctors' income were unrelated to their attitudes toward NHI in 1973. We noted that a similar pattern was found with respect to their expectations and attitudes toward Medicare through 1970; but a strong relationship had emerged by 1973, eight years after Medicare was passed.

17. The problem of "regression" in a longitudinal analysis of conditions (or "qualifiers") under which people do or do not change has been raised by a number of investigators (Hovland, Lumsdaine, and Sheffield, 1949: 329–340; Maccoby, 1956; and Campbell and Clayton, 1961). What is "regression?"

Let us assume no change in the marginal distributions in attitude toward Medicare between Time 1 and Times 2, 3. (The argument holds where there is a large change, as found, but the exposition is clearer if we assume no change.) Let us further assume that individual changes are due entirely to measurement error. If the marginals remain the same, then the *number* of favor-to-oppose changers (call them "+−") must be exactly the same as the number of −+ changers. The *proportions* of those in each initial category would also be equal if the original distribution was 50/50. But the greater the deviation of the marginal distribution from 50/50, the greater will be the *proportion* of those in the initial minority category switching to the majority category, that is, the greater will be the regression effect from the minority to the majority position. (This is the same as "regression to the mean," with the mean of a dichotomous characteristic being the larger proportion.) Thus, a 20 percent positive, 80 percent negative distribution will have a much stronger regression effect from positive to negative than a 45 percent positive, 55 percent negative distribution. The negative-to-positive effect, however, will be stronger in the second distribution than in the first distribution. These results would be obtained assuming no *real* differences in the propensity to change among the various subgroups. (Regression is more apparent intuitively when dealing with continuous variables, e.g., height, weight, or a test score, than with dichotomous characteristics. Its application to the latter is clearly explained in Hovland, Lumsdaine, and Sheffield [1949: 329–340].)

Now if we use as a qualifier variable something that is *related* to attitude toward Medicare at Time 1, this means that the distribution of attitude toward Medicare at Time 1 is different for different values of that qualifier variable. For example, at Time 1, 60 percent of the Democrats favored Medicare, compared with only 15 percent of the Republicans. Hence the regression of the oppose–favor changers is much stronger among the Democrats (40-60) than among the Republicans (85-15). The regression of the favor–oppose changers will of course be stronger among the Republicans than among the Democrats. It follows that the more strongly related party preference is to attitude toward Medicare at Time 1, the larger will be the difference in the regression patterns of Democrats and Republicans. It is this very difference in regression patterns that is confounded with our prediction that Democrats opposed to Medicare at Time 1 were more likely to change than Republicans.

A number of solutions to the problem of regression have been suggested:

(1) Maccoby suggests a retest within a short time to obtain a measure of test-retest reliability. This measure of error could then be subtracted from the change over a longer period of time. The difference between the long-term change and the short-term change ("error") is "real change."

(2) A second approach, recommended by Hovland, is to add a control group—a group

not exposed to the experimental variable. A before-after analysis of the individual cells of this group would indicate the results to be expected due to causes *other* than the experimental variable. Among these other causes are the effects of regression due to errors of measurement (Hovland, Lumsdaine, and Sheffield, 1949: 340).

If neither of these procedures is appropriate for solving the problem of regression in this analysis, does this then mean that the effects of certain qualifier variables in accounting for differential change, as presented here, are vulnerable in that they can be explained away by regression effects? Not necessarily. Consider the following argument:

Not all the qualifier variables in our analysis "worked," that is, differentiated the changers from the nonchangers. Furthermore, some of the qualifier variables that did not work among some subgroups were strongly related to attitude toward Medicare at Time 1, for example, political party in New York City. It is not plausible to argue that regression operates among some subgroups but not among others.

The fact that many of the negative results in our analysis of qualifier variables were not consistent with the operation of regression effects where they would be most expected, that is, where the qualifier variables were strongly related to initial attitudes toward Medicare, suggests that the amount of error in the measurement of attitude toward Medicare at Time 1 is negligible. Substantive interpretations of positive results are thereby strengthened.

18. We examined and tried out a number of approaches exploiting more fully our panel design in order to link changes in the attitudes of individuals toward Medicare with subsequent changes in their attitudes toward other issues. For example, we computed various measures of "mutual effects" and "cross-lagged correlations" (Lazarsfeld, 1947, 1971, 1978; Campbell, 1963; Pelz and Andrews, 1964; Yee and Gage, 1968), but the results were inconclusive. In some cases we obtained opposite results from two different indices of mutual effects, Campbell's cross-lagged panel correlation (with Kendall's tau) and Pelz and Andrews' cross-lagged partial. Our skepticism was reinforced by a paper by Rogers (1967). In a comparison of four different indices of mutual effects computed for 31 tables from fourteen studies, Rogers found that the four indices agreed as to the direction of the effect, that is, in their identification of the stronger variable, in only two-thirds of the tables. We were further cautioned about the appropriateness of using mutual effects methods when there was such a large shift in one of the variables (i.e., attitude toward Medicare).

We also inspected a 64-fold table (attitude toward Medicare and another variable, both dichotomized, at three points in time: $2^3 \times 2^3 = 64$ cells) by arranging the eight patterns of response in attitude toward Medicare at three points in time—Time 1, Times 2, 3 (combined), and Time 4—along one axis and the eight patterns of response to the second item at the same three points in time on the other axis; and examined the data as a contingency table. We did indeed find that the patterns of response on Medicare and those on the second question, for example, of whether "it is the responsibility of the entire society . . . to provide everyone with the best available medical care, whether he can afford it or not" were *correlated* in the expected direction, but knotty questions remained about "causality."

19. In terms of these conditions, the poor prospects of the plan that physicians struck against in Saskatchewan in 1962 could, at least in retrospect, have been predicted: (1) the plan's impact on physicians' practice was much greater than Medicare's, providing for universal coverage for all residents in the province and a comprehensive range of services; (2) public opposition to the plan appeared to be stronger and better organized than the opposition to Medicare; and (3) it was a provincial, not a national plan (Badgley and Wolfe, 1967).

Outside the area of medical care, public response in many parts of the country to statutes and judicial decisions requiring the desegregation of schools and other institutions contrasted sharply with the response of physicians to Medicare. We do not want to compare Medicare and desegregation in any great detail, but some analytic differences between them come to mind: (1) Despite the "American creed" and trends showing a reduction of prejudice and discrimination, at least up to 1964, racism may have been more firmly entrenched among large segments of the Americn public than was the fear of government participation in health care among physicians. (2) The distribution of opposition to desegregation and to Medicare was different: social supports to segregationists were more widely available than social supports to physicians opposed to Medicare. The general public strongly supported Medicare, and it was the medical profession that was out of step. (3) Desegregation, like Medicaid, ran into a hodgepodge of inconsistent and contradictory local, state, and federal laws concerning different facilities and institutions—schools, transportation, recreation, housing, employment, marriage. Some of these laws actually *prescribed* segregation.

7 Does Organized Medicine Represent the Medical Profession?

We began this book by observing that the structure and policies of organized medicine have been the subject of considerable study (Garceau, 1941; "The American Medical Association . . . ," 1954; Burrow, 1963; Freymann, 1964; Harris, 1966; Rayack, 1967; Tatalovich, 1971; Cafferata, 1974; Campion, 1984) compared with the attitudes and perceptions of the nation's rank-and-file physicians. In the preceding chapters we have focused on the latter. We now turn to the question: Does organized medicine represent the medical profession?

The policy positions of organized medicine are generally viewed as more conservative than the opinions of the nation's individual physicians. Nearly 30 years ago, President Harry Truman, writing in his memoirs about the defeat of his national health insurance proposals, said that organized medicine did not represent the true feelings of rank-and-file physicians but of "a small group of men who professed to speak for them and who promoted lobbying by medical organizations to further their own interests" (1956: 20).

A few years later, Dr. Caldwell B. Esselstyn, President of Group Health Association, testifying at a congressional committee hearing on Medicare legislation, said:

> I am here unofficially representing the increasingly substantial number of doctors throughout the country—whose voice has never been heard because of the absence of an effective forum within the American Medical Association where dissenting opinion may be expressed. This has come about because of the basic structure of the AMA, in which democratic rule ends at the county level. . . . Today so-called organized medicine speaks for only a fraction of the physicians in the country—probably the smallest fraction in the last fifteen years. (U.S. Congress, 1961)

Others have concluded that AMA policies do generally reflect the views of the profession (Garceau, 1941: 131–137; "The American Medical Association . . . ," 1954: 947; Rayack, 1967: 16–17).[1] There is little systematic evidence, however, to support either of these positions. Moreover, the question of congruence between the policies of "organized medicine" and the views of individual physicians is complex and the answer is likely to be highly differentiated. In this chapter we compare leaders at the AMA level and leaders, members, and nonmembers at the state and county medical society levels with respect to:

1. their personal and professional characteristics;
2. their attitudes toward political and health care issues; and
3. the degree to which they *feel* represented by the AMA ("subjective representation") and whether they think that dissident physicians should work within the AMA to change it or work with another organization.

But it would be useful to locate these questions within a broader context of interrelated questions by explicating the more general question: "Does organized medicine represent the medical profession?" A part of this explication refers to Michels's classic analysis of characteristics of organizations that lead to oligarchy (1915). We begin by examining the terms "organized medicine," "represent," and "the medical profession."

Organized Medicine. To begin with, we must distinguish between the American Medical Association and its constituent state and county medical societies from a wide variety of other organizations of physicians, including specialty societies, the American College of Physicians, the American College of Surgeons, the Association of American Medical Colleges; and from such organizations as the National Medical Association (black physicians) and the American Medical Women's Association.

The emergence of specialty societies and of organizations such as the Association of American Medical Colleges has increasingly challenged in recent years the AMA's claim as *the* "voice of American medicine" (Stevens, 1971; Tatalovich, 1971: 7–12; Cafferata, 1974).[2]

Moreover, although the AMA and its constituent state and local societies are commonly viewed as monolithic,[3] there is much diversity and conflict within and between these levels (Garceau, 1941: 130–165). Describing the disparate positions on the National Health Service Corps bill taken by the AMA's Councils and its staff, Redman characterizes the AMA's response as "remarkably schizoid" and showing "fretful indecisiveness" (1973). (See also "The AMA House of Delegates: Does it really speak for American medicine?" 1971.)

In short, the first step in explicating the general question is to differentiate "organized medicine."

Represents. The term "represents" can have any one of the following meanings:

1. It can mean the extent to which leaders of organized medicine are similar to nonleaders in their objective *professional* and *social characteristics*, such as their main activity (e.g., patient care, teaching, research, administration), worksetting, specialty, income level, geographic region, age, ethnic and religious background, and gender. Implicit in this concern is the assumption that physicians differ in their views and in their self-interests according to these objective characteristics.

2. The term "represents" can mean the extent to which leaders' attitudes or their actions or organizational policies are consistent with (or serve) the real or perceived *interests* of nonleaders.

3. The term "represents" can mean the extent to which leaders' attitudes or their actions or organizational policies are congruent with nonleaders' *attitudes* on given issues.

The measurement of the degree to which the attitudes of leaders and other physicians are in agreement is relatively straightforward. It involves comparing the distributions of responses to specific questions. But a precise assessment of the degree to which organizational policies and physicians' attitudes correspond is more complex. Such an analysis would have to take into account: the problem of matching policy statements, which are often deliberately qualified and ambiguous to accommodate the perceived diversity of members' views, with statistical distributions of responses to necessarily oversimplified questions in opinion surveys; the variation in the *size* of a majority opinion; and the variation in the *importance* of issues, which would need to be weighted in order to arrive at an overall judgment about the degree of congruence between organizational policies and physicians' attitudes.

In considering the extent of congruence between the attitudes of leaders and members, two questions emerge:

a. How is the extent of congruence or its absence to be explained? In a classical study Michels (1915) analyzed the characteristics of organizational life—the superior knowledge of leaders, their control over means of communication, and their skill in politics and member apathy—that, he argued, make oligarchy inevitable. Nearly 50 years later Lipset, Trow, and Coleman (1956) studied the International Typographical Union as an exception to Michels's "iron law of oligarchy" and identified structural characteristics in that organization that facilitated democracy.

It is generally assumed that oligarchy leads to incongruence between the attitudes of leaders and members, whereas democracy leads to congruence. But congruence may be achieved in an oligarchic organization, too. A parroting of leaders' positions by members, without adequate knowledge, discussion, and reflection on the issues may produce a high degree of congruence. According to Garceau, the AMA's organizational media have a strong influence in "molding" the uninformed opinions of physicians (1941: 96–103).

b. If leaders' and members' attitudes are not congruent, what is the *direction* of that difference and how is it to be explained?

One model posits that leaders' attitudes fall between those of their membership and the dominant ideology of the larger society, since one function of leadership is to mediate between the organization and its social environment (Thompson and McEwen, 1958). Michels's (1915) observation that the leadership of the left-of-center German Social Democratic Party were more conservative than the members is consistent with this model. Since rank-and-file physicians are more conservative than the general population (see Chapter 2), we would expect, according to this model, the leadership of organized medicine to be more liberal than its membership on political and health care issues.

A second model posits that leaders' attitudes are more extreme and intense than those of their membership. For example, the views of leaders of the Democratic and Republican parties were found to be further apart than the views of the rank-and-file of the two parties (McClosky, Hoffman, and O'Hara, 1960: 422).

A third logical alternative is that leaders are generally more conservative—or more progressive—than their membership, regardless of the position of the latter's views on the political spectrum.

The Medical Profession. The third term in the original question, "the medical profession," needs to be differentiated, as was "organized medicine." Physicians differ according to their main activity, the organizational setting in which they work, how they are reimbursed, their specialty—and subspecialty—and so on (on professional segments see Bucher and Strauss, 1961, cited earlier). Some of these segments may be better represented by some parts of organized medicine than by others. New organizations are often established, in fact, to represent the special interests of segments of the profession.

With these observations as a framework, we turn to our empirical analysis and compare leaders at the AMA level and leaders, members, and nonmembers at the state and county medical society level with respect to their objective professional and social characteristics, their attitudes toward political and health care issues, and whether they feel represented by the AMA.

Physicians were classified as leaders, members, and nonmembers as follows (see Q's 63 and 65):

1. *AMA leaders*—those who had served as an officer or committee chairperson on the AMA level in the prior five years;
2. *State leaders*—those who had served as an officer or committee chairperson in their state medical society or in both their state and county medical societies, but not at the national, AMA level, in the prior five years;
3. *County leaders*—those who had served as an officer or committee chairperson in their county, but not in their state medical society in the prior five years;
4. *Members*—those who were members of their state and/or county medical society at the time of the interview, but had not held office in either in the prior five years;
5. *Nonmembers*—all other physicians.

Roughly one-fifth (23%) of the sample were identified as "leaders," less than 1 percent (22 physicians) at the AMA level, 7 percent at the state level, and 15 percent at the county level; another two-thirds (63%) were identified as "members" (with state and county membership almost completely overlapping), and about one-seventh (14%) were identified as "nonmembers." Considering the size and nature of the state and county "leader" categories, we view them as "grass-roots leaders."

In addition, for the 236 members of the AMA House of Delegates in 1973, biographical and professional data in the American Medical Directory (1974) were tabulated and included in Table 7-2.

We reemphasize that our four categories of state and county leaders, members, and nonmembers refer only to participation in the state and county medical societies. AMA membership was closely related to these four categories: 90 percent of the state leaders, 88 percent of the county leaders, and 80 percent of the state/county members were also members of the AMA, compared with only 20 percent of the state/county nonmembers. Another way of summarizing overlapping membership on the national, state, and county levels is as follows: two-thirds (69%) were members of the AMA as well as the state and/or county medical society; 17 percent were members of the state and/or county medical societies only; 3 percent of the physicians in our sample were members of the AMA only. This makes a total of 90 percent of the physician sample (including the 22 AMA leaders) who were members of one or more of the following: the AMA, their state medical society, or their county medical society.[4]

Membership in the AMA among senior physicians (i.e., excluding members of housestaffs) has declined from about 72 (69+3) percent in

1973 to about 60 percent in the early eighties; membership in state and/or county medical societies also appears to have declined, but by not as much—from 86 percent to about 80 percent. (Recent estimates are based on computations from the following sources, adjusting for the inclusion of housestaffs and for the major activity groupings among senior physicians: Louis Harris and Associates, 1981: 60–61; American Medical Association, 1981a: 59–60; Louis Harris and Associates, 1984.)

Our classification of leaders, members, and nonmembers was validated by its correlation with reported attendance at medical society meetings and with self-reports of interest and information about health care issues (see Table 7-1). Those in each of the three levels of leadership, not surprisingly, were most likely to have attended at least one meeting in the past year of the society in which they held that office. Leaders were also more interested in health care issues and were better informed about national health insurance (NHI) than were members and nonmembers, the level of interest and information rising with level of leadership.

Findings

Social Background and Professional Characteristics

The extent to which leaders and members are similar in their background characteristics may provide a proxy measure of the ideological congruence between the two groups, as discussed above. Differences in these objective characteristics may provide clues to explain attitudinal differences. On the other hand, leaders and members may be similar in their objective characteristics but different in their attitudes because of selection into, or socialization by, leadership role activities.

These characteristics may also be considered in their own right. Some of them (age, being a male, membership in a majority rather than in a minority ethnic-religious group) may indicate social credentials that facilitate physicians' careers, including careers in medical politics (see Hall, 1946). Some characteristics may indicate opportunities linked to career stage. For example, again consider age. It may be only after a physician has devoted some years to building a practice that he or she can afford to participate in medical society activities. Finally, some characteristics may point to individual interests that are served by being active in the medical society and getting to be known by one's colleagues. For example, specialists in fee-for-service practice may gain, or hope to gain, referrals.

Table 7-1. Attendance at Medical Society Meetings, Interest in Health Care Issues, and Information about NHI by Medical Society Membership and Level of Leadership

	Leaders			Members	Nonmembers
Base N's	AMA (22)	State (193)	County (404)	(1,713)	(384)
Percent who attended any meetings in the past 12 months of:					
County medical society	84	90	95	67	DNA[a]
State medical society	63	90	45	34	DNA
American Medical Association	60	25	14	15	3
Interest in health care issues					
Q. 69. Comparing yourself to most physicians you know, do you take more active interest in issues in the organization of health care, or less active interest, or about the same?					
Percent responding "more active interest"	65	57	29	18	20
Information about NHI					
Q. 21 Different proposals have been made in the past few years for a *national health insurance* plan covering everyone in the population. How well informed do you feel you are about the various proposals? Are you very well informed, or fairly well informed, or not well informed, or not at all informed?.					
Percent responding "very well informed"	46	20	6	6	4

[a]DNA = Does not apply.

Three patterns of differences in the background characteristics of leaders, members, and nonmembers appear in Table 7-2.

One pattern—that of physicians' age—shows a stepwise difference between nonmembers and members and between successive levels of leadership. Our finding that leaders were older than members is consistent with that of other studies (Garceau, 1941: 58–60; Tatalovich, 1971: 66–68); and the progressive increase in age with level of leadership reflects the succession of offices held by leaders as they rise from county to state to national positions. A study of the 1971 House of Delegates, including Alternates, found that the median age of those who attained delegate status was 52 years, following a median of five years spent in positions at the county level, ten years at the state level, and three years as an Alternate ("The AMA House of Delegates . . . ," (1971: 38).

Nonmembers were overrepresented in salaried patient care or in other salaried activities (research, teaching, administration) in part because they were younger (only 30% were over 45); 83 percent were in such salaried positions compared with between one-fifth and one-third of the leaders and members. The benefits of medical society membership—malpractice and other insurance programs, retirement plans, aids in establishing and managing a practice, and the like—are of more interest to private practitioners than they are to salaried practitioners. But young physicians were still less likely to be medical society members, controlling for their main activity and whether they were salaried or not.

A second pattern, involving the social background characteristics of gender, religious upbringing, race, and U.S. generational status, shows members and nonmembers to be generally similar, but different from leaders, with no systematic difference among the latter according to level of leadership. Leaders were slightly more likely to possess "socially preferred" characteristics than were members and nonmembers: they were more likely to be male, Protestant, white, and U.S.-born with U.S.-born parents. Leaders, members, and nonmembers did not differ, however, in their socioeconomic origins.

The degree of urbanization of the places where physicians lived and worked is an exception to this pattern, but it is probably due to an "artifact." Garceau observed, in 1930, when most physicians were from cities and towns with a population of less than 100,000 (31% were from towns of under 5,000), that the AMA and state medical societies "are run by doctors with city backgrounds" (Garceau, 1941: 50–53). In 1973 we found quite the opposite situation: physicians from large metropolitan areas were underrepresented among leaders, especially at the state and county levels, compared with members and nonmembers. (This conclusion is consistent with an analysis of 1960–70 leaders by Tatalovich, 1971:

Table 7-2. Personal and Professional Characteristics by Medical Society Membership and Level of Leadership

	Leaders					
Base N's	AMA House of Delegates (236)[a]	AMA (22)	State (193)	County (404)	Members (1,713)	Nonmembers (384)
NONPROFESSIONAL CHARACTERISTICS						
Age						
Percent over 45	97	85	83	68	58	30
Gender						
Percent male	100[b]	100	98	98	94	92
Religion						
Percent Protestant upbringing	—[c]	62	75	67	46	44
Race						
Percent White	—[c]	100	97	95	94	93
Nativity						
Percent U.S.-born with U.S.-born parents	—[c]	82	78	71	57	62
Socioeconomic Background						
Percent whose fathers were college graduates	—[c]	36	49	40	38	46

170

USMG-FMG						
Percent trained in U.S. medical schools	97	100	96	94	86	84
Urbanization						
Percent in SMSA's of 1 million or over	44	37	25	20	53	64
PROFESSIONAL CHARACTERISTICS						
Salaried	—[c]	34	20	19	26	83
Specialty						
General/family practice	19	23	24	28	20	16
Surgical specialties	42	25	36	28	30	11
Medical specialities	10	22	20	21	21	27
All other specialties[d]	29	30	20	22	29	46
Percent board-certified	60	47	59	48	49	37
Income						
Percent with net professional income $40,000 or more (in 1972)	—[c]	47	55	59	48	10

[a]These data we obtained from the American Medical Directory (American Medical Association, 1974) for all 236 members of the AMA House of Delegates.

[b]Based on first names in American Medical Directory.

[c]Data not available.

[d]Includes anesthesiology, occupational medicine, pathology, psychiatry, public health, radiology, and "others."

68–72.) The difference may be due to differences between Garceau's and our definitions of "urban-rural" and "leadership," or it may be due to the large shift of physicians to large urban centers since the 1930s. Since the number of county and state medical societies and, consequently, the number of offices and committees in these societies, has probably remained relatively stable since 1930 and since societies in rural areas have nearly as many offices and committees as those in more populated ones, urban physicians are necessarily underrepresented among "leaders" at the state and county levels.

The slight upturn of urban physicians in the House of Delegates reflects the house's rule allocating more delegates to those states with the largest number of physicians, which generally include the largest cities. But urban physicians are still underrepresented at the national level.

A third pattern appears when we turn to *professional* characteristics. Leaders were very much like members, and very unlike nonmembers. Most striking was the high proportion of medical society members and leaders who were primarily engaged in fee-for-service patient care, in contrast to nonmembers, who were primarily in salaried positions in patient care, research, teaching, and administration.

In contrast to Garceau's findings in the 1930s (Garceau, 1941: 54–57), however, specialists were not overrepresented among the leaders. Although the proportion of leaders who were general practitioners has dropped since the 1930s, the proportion of nonleaders who were general practitioners has dropped even more.[5]

Associated in part with their concentration in salaried work, specialties such as psychiatry, radiology, pathology, occupational medicine, and public health were overrepresented among nonmembers, while the surgical specialties were underrepresented. Members and leaders, however, were very similar in their specialty distributions.

With respect to their professional income, only 10 percent of the nonmembers earned $40,000 or more, just above the median; and nonmembers were least likely to be board-certified.

Attitudes Toward Political and Health Care Issues

Members tended to be more liberal than leaders, but these differences, although statistically significant, were not strong (Table 7-3); leaders and members were much more similar in their views than expected. In contrast, nonmembers were considerably more liberal than both leaders and members in their political views and in their attitudes toward government-in-medicine and health care issues. There were two exceptions to

Table 7-3. Attitudes toward Political and Health Care Issues by Medical Society Membership and Level of Leadership[a]

	Leaders				Members	Nonmembers
Base N's	AMA (22)	State (193)	County (404)	Total (619)	(1,713)	(384)
Political ideology (% liberal)	26	26	28	27	40	62
"Government-in-medicine" (% liberal)	37	31	33	33	46	66
Group practice (% favor)	22	18	31	27	35	67
Peer reviews (% favor)	59	43	30	35	39	52
Task delegation (% favor)	74	48	40	44	37	56
Physician reimbursement (% accept salaried/capitation)	32	20	22	22	28	51
Prepayment (% accept)	35	46	31	36	41	60

[a]See notes to Table 4-1. As in Tables 4-1, 4-2, and 5-1, the figures in this table show the proportion of physicians in each category who took a "liberal" position on each issue.

All paired comparisons between the mean scores of all leaders (AMA, state, and county leaders, combined) versus members and between members versus nonmembers are significant at the .01 level, except for that between the mean scores on attitudes toward peer reviews of leaders versus members.

this pattern: with respect both to peer reviews and to delegation of tasks, AMA leaders were more progressive in their thinking than any other group.

These relationships hold up controlling for social background and professional characteristics of physicians and AMA membership (AMA members are generally less likely than nonmembers to take liberal positions).[6]

A 1983–84 study of physicians' attitudes shows that physician leaders and a national cross-section of physicians differed in their attitudes toward some issues, notably their attitudes toward the need for changes in our health care system and their satisfaction with the quality of care, the cross-section taking more critical positions. But they were quite similar on most other issues, such as utilization reviews, diagnosis-related groups (DRGs), and HMOs, (Louis Harris and Associates, 1984.) It should be noted, however, that that analysis included in the cross-section both local medical society nonmembers and housestaff, who are more liberal than members. Also, the sampling design of leaders in that study was a bit different from ours—it was drawn from the 1981 AMA directory of officials and staff to represent "the leadership of state, local, and specialty medical societies."

Subjective Representation

Thus far we have examined the question: To what extent were leaders "representative" of local members and nonmembers? We consider next the extent to which physicians felt represented by the AMA. We call this "subjective representation."

These questions are recognized by the organization itself in a brochure with the title, "Does the AMA really represent your interests?" distributed to potential members (American Medical Association, undated [ca. 1975]: 3–6):

> It is obvious that neither the AMA nor, for that matter, any organization can represent all of the doctors all of the time. There is just too much difference of thought and opinion. And this is intensified by a characteristic that most physicians share: that of being strong individualists.

The brochure continues:

> If the AMA didn't speak for the profession, who would? . . . . Who would go before the Committees of Congress to state the professions' views on national health insurance, PSROs, HMOs . . . there is only one organization that can and does effectively speak for the profession as a whole—your AMA.

Do physicians feel represented by the AMA?

Asked if they thought the AMA represented their personal opinion on "issues in the organization of health care," a fifth (20%) of all physicians reported that it does so on "most matters," a fifth (23%) on "hardly any," and slightly more than half (55%) on "some." Responses varied according to both medical society and AMA membership and leadership level. As expected, the degree of feeling represented generally rose, comparing nonmembers with members and county, state, and national leaders, in that order (see Table 7-4) and within each of these categories (with the exception of national leaders, since they are all AMA members), AMA members were more likely to feel represented than AMA nonmembers. Of those who were not members of their county or state societies or the AMA, only 6 percent felt represented on most issues, compared with 38 percent among state leaders who were members of the AMA, and with 48 percent among the AMA leaders.

The point worth noting here is that even among state leaders who were AMA members, less than half (38%)—and among national leaders, barely half (48%)—felt that the AMA represented their personal opinion on "most matters" in health care delivery. Without comparative data about other professions and professional organizations, however, the interpretation of these figures is problematic. Moreover, because of differences in the sampling designs, response rates, and in the wording of questions in other studies of physicians' feelings about being represented by the AMA—before and since our 1973 study—it is difficult to identify trends.[7] It appears, however, that a substantial number of American physicians do not feel represented by the AMA, and that this number has remained generally stable over the past decade.

In any case, when confronted with the question of whether physicians who disagree with AMA policies should work within that organization and try to change it or work with another organization, fully 80 percent thought that dissenting physicians should work within the AMA. Even among those who felt represented on "hardly any" issues, half (52%) supported working with the organization. (Responses to the two questions were highly correlated: among those who felt represented by the AMA on "most" matters, 96% believed that dissenting physicians should work within it.)

On this question, however, the difference in responses according to medical society membership and level of leadership (see Table 7-4) is explained almost entirely by membership in the AMA: between 91 and 99 percent of the AMA members within each of the four main medical society-leadership-membership categories preferred that physicians work within the AMA, while between 52 and 68 percent (note, still no less than

Table 7-4. Feeling Represented and Alternatives to AMA by Medical Society Membership and Level of Leadership

	Leaders			Members	Nonmembers
Base N's	AMA (22)	State (193)	County (404)	(1,713)	(384)
Do physicians feel represented by AMA?					
Q. 67. Thinking about issues in the organization of health care, does the AMA represent your personal opinion on most matters, on some, or on hardly any?					
Percent responding "on most matters"	48	35	25	21	9
Alternatives for physicians who disagree with AMA					
Q. 68. Should doctors who disagree with the policies of the AMA try to change the organization by working within it, or by working with another organization?					
Percent responding "work within"	92	95	88	86	71

half) of the non-AMA members expressed this preference (data not shown).

AMA policies are viewed as too conservative to suit liberal physicians and too liberal to suit conservative physicians. Since AMA policies are perceived as generally conservative,[8] however, it is not surprising that liberal physicians were less likely than conservative physicians to feel represented by the AMA. (For example, 29% of those with the most conservative position on NHI felt represented on "most matters," compared with only 6% of those with the most liberal position.)

In Chapter 2 we discussed physicians' underestimation of their colleagues' support for NHI as an instance of pluralistic ignorance. We speculated that many physicians, not knowing how their colleagues actually felt about NHI, ascribed views to them that were in line with what they *perceived* to be the conservative policies of the AMA; they assumed that the AMA "spoke for" other doctors, if not for themselves.

But, if AMA and medical society leaders' *attitudes* have some general objective correspondence to AMA *policies*, our findings that the attitudes of leaders and members were generally congruent suggest that physicians (including leaders) perceive AMA policies as more conservative than they are in fact. It is noteworthy that even among our small sample of AMA leaders and among those physicians with the most conservative attitudes toward given political and health care issues, fewer than half (Table 7-4) and no more than one-third, respectively, felt represented by the AMA on "most matters."

To explore why the AMA is perceived as more conservative than it is in fact goes beyond the scope of this chapter. But one plausible explanation goes back to our earlier characterization of the AMA and its constituent medical societies as internally differentiated and diverse. For nearly half a century, beginning in the mid-1920s, the ultraconservative views of Morris Fishbein were identified by both physicians and the general public as the "voice" of the AMA. Fishbein's influence and activities extended far beyond his duties as editor of the AMA's *Journal* from 1923 to 1949 (Burrow, 1963: 169–170; Campion, 1984: 113–125).

Although Fishbein's views may never have represented the moderate center of the AMA leadership, that disparity probably increased over time, especially after the passage of Medicare, as the AMA adopted a less obstructive stance on health care issues.[9] Fishbein was relieved of his duties as *Journal* editor in 1949 because he had alienated so many groups both within and outside the profession (Burrow, 1963: 373–374; Campion, 1984: 113–125). An obituary in the *New England Journal of Medicine* stated that "he became too powerful to be tolerated" by the AMA's Board of Trustees ("Morris Fishbein, M.D.," 1976: 1134).

Nevertheless, our argument continues, the AMA is still being remembered as it was before Medicare, when Fishbein and other ultraconservatives were viewed as the organization's official spokesmen. In short, there may be a "reputational lag" between moderate changes in AMA policies (discussed in Chapter 2) and perceptions of these new policies.

Summary

Does organized medicine represent the medical profession? Any answer must take into account the diversity of both physicians and their professional organizations. In summary, we have found the following:

Leaders at the county and state medical society level and at the national AMA level were slightly more likely than both medical society members and nonmembers to possess such "socially preferred" characteristics as being Protestant, born in the United States with U.S.-born parents, male, and white. Leaders were also older than members, their age rising with the level of leadership (county, state, and national); and members were older than nonmembers.

However, leaders were remarkably similar to members in such professional characteristics as whether they were in fee-for-service patient care, their specialty, and their professional income. Moreover, leaders were remarkably similar to members in their attitudes toward a range of political and health care issues such as the role of government-in-medicine, group practice, peer reviews, the delegation of tasks, salaried reimbursement to physicians, and prepayment.

In contrast, leaders and members differed sharply from nonmembers in their professional characteristics and in their attitudes. Nonmembers were more likely than leaders and members to be salaried; to be in such specialties as psychiatry, radiology, pathology, occupational medicine, and public health, rather than in surgery; to earn lower incomes; and to hold liberal opinions.

In a word, leaders appeared to speak for their membership, but not for that part of the profession who do not join their county and state medical societies—mainly salaried practitioners, teachers, administrators, and researchers. In view of the growing number of physicians working in salaried settings, these leaders may be speaking in the future for a progressively shrinking segment of the profession.

Although physicians felt, at best, only moderately represented by the AMA (only a fifth reported that the AMA represented their personal opinion on "most matters" in the organization of health care), the majority (80%) felt that physicians who disagreed with AMA policies should "try to change the organization by working within it" rather than "[work] with another organization."

That physicians with liberal opinions on political and health care issues were less likely to feel represented by the AMA than those with conservative opinions is consistent with the general perception of AMA policies as being more conservative than the general level of physician opinion. What accounts for this perception?

We speculated that despite adaptations in AMA policies in recent decades, especially since the passage of Medicare, to bring these policies more closely in line with prevailing nonmedical—and physician—opinion, there has been a "lag" in physicians' *perceptions* of these policy changes. Thus, although AMA policies might, in fact, be more congruent with the opinions of physicians than they were two or three decades ago, they are perceived as being less congruent than they actually are.

Thus, whereas, on the one hand, the legitimacy of the AMA's claim as spokesman for the entire profession is undermined by a declining membership and a growing differentiation of segments with their own special interest societies and organizations, on the other hand, that claim is supported by evidence of a closer alignment than is commonly believed between AMA policies and the opinions of a still sizeable number of physicians on salient and important issues.

Notes

1. It should be noted that Rayack qualifies his conclusion by observing that the AMA reflects the will of the "overwhelming majority of physicians *in private medical practice*" (*Emphasis added*).

2. These challenges were recognized by a former president of the AMA, at the same time reasserting the AMA's dominant role as spokesman of the profession:

> At one time [the AMA's] preeminence was apparent to anyone who would look. In some respects it may be less towering and less visible today, not because of any diminution of its own stature, but because, as a part of the great growth in medicine and its specialties, there has been *an emergence of other organizations*—in surgery, in medicine, in family practice, and on through the roster. Still and all, while sharing with others the ever more difficult task of exerting leadership in the pure science of medicine, the AMA has remained the bastion of professionalism and the stronghold of responsible socioeconomic leadership. ("This is the AMA," 1973: 139) (*Emphasis added*)

3. A 1955 survey found that nearly three-quarters of the public and one-half of physicians perceived "no difference" between the AMA and its constituent state and county societies (Gaffin, 1956: 40).

4. We also examined overlapping memberships and leadership positions across two broad types of professional organizations: those consisting of the AMA and its constituent state and county medical societies ("Type A"); and those consisting of all other physicians' organizations ("Type B"). The latter are dominated by specialty societies, but they are extremely heterogeneous, including such organizations as the American Medical Women's Association, the National Medical Association (primarily black physicians), and the politically liberal Physicians' Forum.

We find a fair amount of overlapping *memberships* across the two types of organizations, but only a limited number of overlapping *leaderships*. The majority (73%) of all physicians belong to both types of organizations. Among those reporting holding office or chairing a committee in *any* organization, however (a third of all physicians), only one-fifth (19%) held positions *both* in Type A medical societies and in Type B professional associations. (Even this may be an overestimate, since the interview question asked if the respondent had been an officer or committee chairman in "the past five years." Hence, some of these overlapping leadership positions may in fact not have been held simultaneously.)

5. Tatalovich (1971: 56–61) found that the distribution of specialists and general practitioners varied according to level and office held: GP's were strongly overrepresented among county medical society presidents in 1970, probably due in part to the geographic artifact mentioned above, and the distribution among state medical society presidents was quite similar to that among the AMA House of Delegates, but surgeons were even more overrepresented and general practitioners underrepresented among the top AMA officers, including President, Executive Vice-President, Secretary-Treasurer, Speaker of the House of Delegates, and members of the Board of Trustees and of key councils.

6. We expected the *degree* of congruence between leaders and members to vary according to the content and specificity of the issue area examined: namely, that leaders and members would be in closer agreement on the more concrete and specific health care issues, such as NHI, group practice, peer reviews, and method of reimbursement, on which the AMA has taken policy positions, than on the more general, nonhealth, ideological areas such as economic-welfare liberalism, political party preference, and general political identity, on which the AMA has taken either less explicit policy positions or no positions at all. We thought this pattern would indicate the mutual influence between AMA policies and physicians' attitudes. However, there was no clear pattern of intergroup differences in attitudes according to issue area.

We also checked to see if there was an AMA "party line" among successive levels of leadership and participation in organized medicine. We expected that such a party line would be strongest among state leaders and weakest among nonmembers. Operationally, we expected interstate variation in physicians' attitudes toward political and health care issues to increase among state leaders, county leaders, members, and nonmembers, in that order. The absence of such a pattern—that is, if the amount and pattern of interstate variation were the same among state leaders, county leaders, members, and nonmembers—would suggest that local leaders are more representative and responsive to their local constituencies than they are followers of a central AMA party line. With respect to NHI, the one issue we examined this way, our data do not support the presence of a party line.

7. In a 1955 survey, three-fourths (77%) of the private practitioners interviewed said that "AMA policies satisfied most doctors." On the other hand, half (49%) thought the AMA was run by only "a few doctors" (Gaffin, 1956: 23–25); in a 1970 survey of hospital interns, residents, and salaried staff and academic physicians (on the basis of only a 25% response rate), 63 percent said that the AMA speaks for the medical profession ("Where doctors stand . . . ," 1970); and in a Harris survey reported in 1970, roughly a third (38%) responded

"yes," a third (36%), "no," and a quarter (26%) gave a qualified answer to the question: "Does the American Medical Association accurately represent your views on most professional matters?" ("What doctors think of their patients," 1970). Finally, in an AMA-sponsored survey in 1981 in which physicians were asked how often the AMA represented their views on a number of issues (NHI, HMOs, second opinions, abortion), their responses were closer to "usually" than to "occasionally," based on average scores derived from ratings of "practically never," "occasionally," "usually," and "almost always" (American Medical Association, 1981: 62–63).

8. The AMA acknowledges this in the brochure addressed to prospective members: "The majority of people think of the AMA as a conservative organization." And then attempts to modify this image: "It does have its share of conservatives. But it also has its share of liberals and middle-of-the-roaders" (American Medical Association, undated [ca. 1975]: 2). The fact remains, however, that even members of the House of Delegates, as we noted in Chapter 2, perceived the House as more conservative than themselves ("The AMA House of Delegates: Does it really speak for American medicine?" 1971: 39).

9. For an excellent analysis of changes in the AMA as a case study of bureaucratic adaptation to external social pressures, see Tatalovich (1971). For an analysis of earlier shifts, in the early 1920s, in the composition of the AMA's leadership (from academicians to private practitioners) and in its policies (from progressive to conservative), see Freymann (1964).

8 Summary and Conclusions

In this concluding chapter, we summarize our main findings on the attitudes of physicians toward political and health care issues and our conceptual framework of socialization in relation to these findings. We also review briefly the major events on the political and health care scene since the mid-seventies, when our data were collected. Then we discuss the implications of our findings on the attitudes of physicians for health care, first, by outlining a framework for establishing the general relevance of these attitudes for health care policies and programs, and, second, by linking findings from our research and from more recent studies of these attitudes to current and emerging issues. This discussion is based on our conviction that the practical value of social science research findings is enhanced to the extent that they are generated and grounded in a conceptual framework that transcends narrowly concrete and topical issues.

Summary of Findings
Attitudes Toward Political and Health Care Issues

The medical profession is often portrayed as monolithically conservative, resistant to political change and to modifications in the organization of health care. This, we found, is a misleading caricature. Not only do physicians vary among themselves in their views but they also discriminate among different features and aspects of a set of issues (Chapter 2).

- Although more conservative politically than the general population,

substantial portions of physicians held liberal views: one-fourth considered themselves "liberal" in their political thinking, slightly more than a third, "middle-of-the-road"; one-third were Democrats.
- Considerable numbers supported a role for government in health care, the level of support varying according to specifics; indeed, a majority favored "some form" of national health insurance.
- Some favored and others opposed group practice, the levels depending on specifying which types of group practice; more than half considered a "small" group practice as most desirable, compared to a fourth who chose a "large" group.
- Over 80 percent favored peer reviews in hospitals, about 50 percent even in doctors' offices; three-quarters favored peer reviews under national health insurance.
- Two-thirds would have used a nurse-practitioner or physician's assistant in their practice, but they were much more willing to delegate some tasks than others.
- Fixed fees under NHI were acceptable to nearly two-thirds, capitation to a fourth, and salary to 14 percent.

Physicians underestimated the support of their colleagues for some form of national health insurance—a clear instance of "pluralistic ignorance," when individuals assume that they are virtually alone in holding a certain attitude, not knowing that others privately share it. Why are physicians as a group perceived both by physicians themselves and by the general public to be more conservative than they are in fact? We suggested that both groups, lacking other sources of information, attributed to the profession as a whole the historically conservative policies of the AMA.

The attitudes of physicians toward issues in the organization and delivery of health care, especially toward those issues that explicitly involve the participation of government, were indeed associated with their political views. Health care issues thus are highly politicized; they are not solely "professional" or "scientific" issues, as claimed by some medical spokesmen, who seek to "keep politics out of health."

Social and Professional Characteristics in Relation to Attitudes

Except for their socioeconomic origins, the social background characteristics of physicians, notably their religious upbringing, had a strong effect on their political and government-in-medicine views (Chapter 4). The findings were typical of those in the general population: Jews, women, those who were first-generation, easterners, and urbanites all held more liberal views than did Catholics and Protestants, men, those who were second- and third-or-more-generation, noneasterners, and non-urbanites. We explained the absence of a relationship between the socio-economic origins of physicians and their political views, in sharp contrast to typical findings in the general population, in terms of social selection into medicine from different socioeconomic backgrounds: physicians barely differed in their political views according to their socioeconomic origins when they entered medical school.

Conversely, whereas the social background characteristics of physicians were unrelated to their health care views (group practice, peer reviews, task delegation, physician reimbursement, and prepayment), their professional characteristics ("worksetting" and, to a lesser extent, specialty), viewed as sources of later socialization, influenced both their health care views and their political and government-in-medicine views.

On all issues, physicians in individual, fee-for-service practice were generally the most conservative, followed in declining order by those in (1) group or hospital-based, fee-for-service practice, (2) group or hospital-based, salaried practice, and (3) those whose main activity was teaching, administration, or research rather than patient care.

Considering specialty differences, general practitioners and surgeons were the most conservative on political and government-in-medicine issues, and psychiatrists the most liberal. Those in the medical specialties, including pediatrics, were in between. Our attempt to explain these interspecialty differences in attitudes in terms of specific attributes of the specialties—their prestige and average income and the degree of interaction between practitioner and patient—did not show any meaningful results. Clearly, *why* physicians in different specialties vary in their views remains an intriguing question.

Ideology Across Generations and Changes Due to "Period" Effects

The ideology of the medical profession is not frozen in time. It may change as older generations of physicians are replaced by younger physicians (Chapter 5). And it may change as the profession as a whole adapts to changes in the political and health care systems.

Generational differences were tied to specific sets of policy issues and depended on how broadly "generations" were defined. The much-publicized "generation gap" between medical students and housestaff and their professional elders in the late sixties and early seventies was limited to political and government-in-medicine issues. Moreover, that liberal shift among medical trainees appears to have been short-lived: by the mid-1970s they were more conservative than their predecessors in the early 1970s.

The turbulent events of the sixties obscured the impact of less visible and more glacierlike, but potentially more significant and enduring, changes in the organization of health care in the decades preceding the sixties, changes that have left their mark on the views of successive, more broadly defined generations of physicians. Those who entered practice after Medicare were much more willing than those who entered before World War II to accept group practice, peer reviews, and the delegation of tasks. These generations differed little, or not at all, however, with respect to political and government-in-medicine issues or with respect to salaried, capitation, and fixed-fee reimbursement and prepayment.

The dramatic accommodation of physicians, in thinking and deed, to the passage and implementation of Medicare (but not to Medicaid in New York State) exemplifies another source of change. The attitudes of the profession as a whole were transformed by a relatively specific and concrete event, in this case, the enactment of a governmentally financed health care payment plan (Chapter 6).

The sharp change in the attitudes of physicians toward Medicare "rubbed off" on their attitudes toward some closely related issues—notably, acceptance of the principle of health care as a right, of a greater role for the federal government in the field of health, and of the inadequacy of medical care for poor people. Untouched, however, were their attitudes toward Medicaid, their general political ideology, their attitudes toward general economic-welfare issues and the relatively apolitical health care issues of group practice, peer reviews, and task delegation.

Does Organized Medicine Represent the Medical Profession?

The views of leaders at the AMA, state, and county medical society level were remarkably in tune with those of their membership (Chapter 7). But the *non*members, the 14 percent of all physicians in 1973 (excluding housestaffs) who belonged to neither their state or county medical societies, were much more liberal on most political and health care issues.

Who were these nonmembers? They were younger, they earned lower incomes, and they were much more likely than both leaders and members to be in salaried positions in patient care, research, teaching, and administration. In view of the growing number of physicians in salaried settings, the leadership of organized medicine may be speaking in the future for a smaller and smaller segment of the profession.

Socialization Theory and Professional Attitudes:
A Conceptual Framework

Both *diversity* and *change* in physicians' attitudes toward political and health care issues were analyzed in terms of lifelong *socialization*. Social and professional characteristics, at various stages in the life cycle, were viewed as indicators of socially patterned experiences that influence attitudes. Attitudinal differences between generations of medical trainees and physicians pointed to the influence of broadly defined historical events, translated, again, as (socially) patterned experiences. Finally, a specific historical event, the passage and implementation of Medicare, was viewed as an event experienced by the profession as a whole and as having a dramatic impact on its attitudes toward that relatively circumscribed issue.

Balancing the earlier emphasis on childhood experiences and their presumed lasting impact on lifelong attitudes and values, we have noted the growth of research interest in the last decade or two in adult socialization and in socialization through the life cycle. With particular reference to professionals, it has been argued that with lengthier and increasingly more intensive professional training, the effects of early background on the attitudes, behavior, and careers of individuals are obliterated. Others have taken the argument one step further. They point out that even the effects of professional training fade in the face of the immediate pressures of the current social setting of work. Our findings do, indeed, substantiate the impact of the latter on current attitudes.

But our findings also indicate that, with respect to some types of attitudes, the effects of early, nonprofessional sources of socialization cannot be summarily dismissed. Differences in the political views of sociodemographic groups entering the profession correspond, with some exceptions, to differences in the views of those groups in the general population, and moreover, these differences persist over time. Clearly, the relative impact of early nonprofessional and of later professional sources of socialization depends on the domain of the attitudes. Early and nonprofessional sources generally have a strong effect on attitudes toward more diffuse issues, such as broad political leanings, and practically none on narrower health care issues; later and professional sources influence attitudes toward both political and health care issues. The extension of this general conceptual framework to research on a wider range of sources of socialization and to attitudes toward a wider range of issues (e.g., practice styles, utilization rates, and ethical issues) would add greatly to understanding of the socialization of professionals.

That physicians differed strongly in both their past and current political views according to their religious and ethnic background, like their counterparts in the general population, but not according to their socioeconomic origins, highlights the effects of *social selection* "out of" a status of origin and the problem of establishing temporal links between sources of socialization and attitudes. Whereas initial political differences among Protestant, Catholic, and Jewish physicians persisted, perhaps because these differences were reinforced by their continuing identification with those groups, even the dim differences among entering physicians from different socioeconomic origins faded, as though blurred by the experiences in their current and new (for some) socioeconomic status.

In the preceding chapters we have raised a number of other conceptual and methodological issues and set a busy agenda for future work: for example, the conceptual and empirical blurring of generational and period effects; the extension of the effects of fait accompli (i.e., the perception of the irreversibility of an event that has taken place) to apply to an event that has not yet taken place—an *anticipatory* fait accompli (i.e., the perception of an event's inevitability); the generalization of attitude change why some attitudes in a structure are affected by an initial change, while others are not; and the effects of prior experiences (e.g., with Medicare) on responses to subsequent programs (e.g., to NHI).

These questions all refer back in a general way to the concept of socialization. But we have also introduced throughout the book the notion of self-interest to interpret certain findings. Clearly, a more precise formulation of socialization, ideology, and self-interest in relation to each other and to people's attitudes toward specific issues would be a major advance.

Politics and Health Care since the Mid-Seventies: Continuity and Change

In describing the context of our 1973 physician survey, we identified (in Chapter 2) the main health care issues leading in to the 1970s, that is, the components of the "crisis" in health care as they were perceived at the time—cost, accessibility, and quality. We went on to describe the longer-term trends in the organization of health care: differentiation and specialization, the bureaucratization of medical practice, salaried reimbursement of physicians, third-party payment for health care, reviews and controls of medical practice, and an increasing role of government in health care.

It would be simplistic to view the recent changes in public and private concerns about health care in this country as having replaced the concerns of a decade ago. Rather current issues have evolved from past issues; some are, in fact, a direct continuation of earlier ones.[1] On the other hand, it would be naive to discuss the policy implications of our analysis without taking into account events that have taken place since the mid-seventies. The adaptation of physicians to Medicare stands as a cautionary example of how they may change their minds rather dramatically within a short period as the result of specific events.

Decline of the Welfare State?

The country entered the 1970s on a wave of "agitation and reform." (This and the next section, An Evolving Health Care Sector, draw on Starr [1982: 379–449], among others.) Undergirded by an expanding economy, demands for a more equitable distribution of the nation's resources were translated into programs to provide better nutrition, decent housing, a more comprehensive system of income maintenance, and wider access to education and health care. Ensuring equitable access to care dominated the health policy agenda: national health insurance appeared inevitable. The political debate over regulatory initiatives such as PSRO's and Certificate of Need as well as government support for Health Maintenance Organizations assumed that these programs would play a role in constraining costs under national health insurance. This period was the context of our 1973 physician survey.

Conflict over national health insurance centered not on *whether*, but on what *type* of program should be enacted. In late 1974, Carl Albert, the Speaker of the House of Representatives, declared that NHI would be the first order of business when Congress reconvened and predicted passage by June, 1975 (*New York Times*, Nov. 23, 1974, p. 34). Senator Edward Kennedy, the leader of liberal forces in the NHI struggle, had joined Representative Wilbur Mills, the powerful chairman of the Ways and Means Committee, in cosponsoring a bill that matched the Nixon administration proposal in most important respects. But the momentum toward passage ground to a halt with the Watergate crisis and the scandal that concluded Representative Mills's political career. Despite some discussion of national health insurance during the Ford and Carter administrations, the issue was clearly languishing.

No longer viewed as a solution to the perceived crises of access and of cost and quality of care, national health insurance became widely regarded as costly and utopian. Although public opinion polls continued to show strong levels of support for NHI throughout the 1970s (see American Medical Association, 1981b; Steiber and Ferber, 1981; Ladd, 1983; Navarro, 1983), they also revealed concern about excessive government expenditures. The political momentum for enacting national health insurance had died. In response to a deepening economic recession and soaring inflation related to the worldwide energy crisis, welfare-state policies came under attack in the United States and throughout advanced capitalist societies (Dowling, 1981). Social programs could no longer be painlessly financed through budgetary surpluses. Social welfare expenditures by all levels of government had grown from $22 billion in 1900 to $428 billion in 1979, which represented an increase from 10.5 to 18.5 percent of the GNP (Berki, 1983: 232).

The expanding regulatory structure of the welfare state also came under increasingly harsh attack. Critics from the political right attacked a wide range of health and safety regulations as ineffective or inefficient. Multifaceted regulatory reforms such as utilization review by PSRO's and limits on hospital capital expansion provided through the Certificate of Need (CON) program were evaluated on the narrow grounds of cost containment and judged a failure.

An alternative solution to the cost dilemma, the market-competition approach, began to attract attention in the late 1970s. Growing out of an economic critique of regulation aimed at the providers of medical care, the market-competition strategy would attempt to restore the price sensitivity of consumers. Proponents argue that to the extent that comprehensive insurance benefits reduce the consumers' out-of-pocket costs, consumers have little incentive to choose less costly over more costly types of care or to refrain from using services of marginal benefit. The specific steps that were advocated include reducing or eliminating federal tax subsidies for health insurance and increasing consumer cost-sharing through mechanisms such as increasing coinsurance. Market-competition strategists also seek to promote the growth of HMO's and other alternative delivery systems. As more efficient and less costly forms of care, alternative systems presumably spur price competition with other providers. According to advocates of this approach, unleashing the competitive forces of the economic market would permit elimination of much of the "burdensome" regulation now in effect. Not surprisingly, the market-competition approach was embraced by political conservatives and became the centerpiece of the conservative agenda for health care reform. (For a more complete explanation of procompetitive reforms, see among others: Enthoven, 1980; Olson, 1981; Havighurst, 1982; and Ricardo-Campbell, 1982. A critical assessment of these proposals is provided by Ginzberg, 1981, Reinhardt, 1982; Roemer, 1982; and Wlodkowski, 1983.)

An Evolving Health Care Sector

The lines of the debate had been drawn, but a consensus behind either liberal or conservative reforms failed to emerge during the late seventies. Meanwhile the context of the debate, the health care delivery and financing system, was undergoing certain developments with implications for the choices confronting not only physicians, but society as a whole. While health economists were prescribing the enactment of procompetitive reforms as the needed antidote to burgeoning health care costs, the health care sector was already becoming much more competitive. The growth in comprehensive insurance benefits, including the enactment of Medicaid and Medicare, set the stage for large-scale corporate investment in health care delivery, notably in for-profit hospital chains. Corporate-owned hospitals, nursing homes, psychiatric hospitals, HMO's, and ambulatory care and hemodialysis centers make up what has been labeled the "new medical-industrial complex" (Relman, 1980; Wohl, 1984). Although large corporations have long been active in the production of pharmaceuticals and medical equipment and supplies, and even proprietary hospitals are not new in American medicine, distinctions are generally drawn between these commercial concerns and those belonging to the new corporate chains. For the first time, decisions directly affecting patient care are being centralized in corporate headquarters.

The transformation of the health care delivery system extends beyond the increasing role of investor-owned corporations. Cost containment efforts have reduced government subsidies for the capital expansion and replacement of hospitals while traditional sources of philanthropic financing have also diminished. Voluntary hospitals in urban areas have particularly experienced a capital-financing squeeze. In 52 large cities, the number of voluntary hospitals declined during the 1970–80 period and thus reversed the trend of the past 50 years (Demkovich, 1982). The growth of alternative sites of care such as HMO's and freestanding surgical and emergency care centers also pose competitive threats to hospitals (Goldsmith, 1981). In an increasingly constricted financial environment, nonprofit hospitals have turned to new types of organizational arrangements, which bear a strong resemblance to those of their for-profit competitors. Nonprofit hospitals are entering management contracts with corporate hospital chains, diversifying into new forms of services, and forming their own multi-institutional hospital systems. The downward pressure on health care costs within an increasingly complex, competitive health care sector has created a demand for more businesslike management practices: the line between the investor-owned and nonprofit hospitals sectors has begun to blur.

Multi-institutional hospital chains grew from roughly 5 percent of all community hospitals in 1965 to over 30 percent in 1981. About 40 percent of such hospitals (28% of beds) are owned or managed by investor-owned companies. Although controlling a relatively small share of all hospital beds, 8.8 percent in 1980, the rate of growth has been fastest in the investor-owned sector (Zuckerman, 1983). (For a more detailed description of the "diversification" and "corporate rationalization" of the health care sector, see Relman, 1980; Goldsmith, 1981; Zuckerman, 1983; Iglehart, 1984; and Wohl, 1984).

A number of analysts observe that the growth of the "new medical-industrial complex" will have profound implications for physician autonomy (Relman, 1980; Starr, 1982; Wohl, 1984) It is clear that in both profit and nonprofit hospital settings the need for greater efficiency has augmented the power of hospital management vis-à-vis medical staffs with ramifications for clinical independence and professional values. Management controls are further enhanced by the prospective payment system based on "Diagnosis Related Groups" (DRG's) adopted for the federal Medicare program in 1983. Organization of hospital expenditures according to DRG's allows identification of physicians whose case management results in nonreimbursable expenditures. In the future, hospital admitting privileges may be limited to physicians with "acceptable" levels of resource use (Spivey, 1984).

Physician dominance within the health care system will almost certainly be affected by a second important trend: their own growing numbers. Largely through government programs that subsidized medical training during the 1960s and 1970s, the physician population ratio rose from 140 doctors per 100,000 population in 1950 to 180 per 100,000 in 1980. The ranks of physicians will continue to expand throughout this decade, with projections for 1990 in the range of 240 per 100,000 (Ginzberg, 1983b). Whether this growing number of physicians entails a "physician surplus" depends to some degree on the assumptions of the analyst: estimates of both demand and supply factors are controversial (Reinhardt, 1982; Ginzberg, 1983b). Physicians in the 1980s and beyond, however, are expected increasingly to confront a "buyer's market." With job applicants outnumbering the jobs that are available, it is unlikely that the medical profession will declare war on new forms of organization or financing based on ideological grounds. Despite ominous rumblings within the medical profession about conflicts with professional values, it does not appear that job openings in corporate chains or salaried practices will go short of applicants. The expanding physician supply is expected to feed the competitive pressures already building within the health care system. (For a further analysis of this issue, see Fuchs, 1981; Ginzberg, et al, 1981; Ginzberg, 1983b).

A New Direction for Public Policy

The elections of 1980 elected a President whose long-term health policy goals were conditioned by "market principles," including increased competition within the health care system. The ideological stalemate in health care and social welfare policy as a whole appeared to be broken, and along with it, the twenty-year commitment to welfare state programs and policies. However, the four-year record of the Reagan administration does not substantiate a decisive social policy reversal. Large-scale cuts in nondefense spending have only stemmed the growth of federal health and social welfare expenditures. Furthermore, much of the funding withdrawn by the federal government from social programs has been replaced by state treasuries (*New York Times,* June 10, 1984, p. 1). This is not to deny that federal cutbacks have had sizeable effects on individual programs and recipients. Individuals dropped from the welfare rolls because of narrowed eligibility criteria have also lost Medicaid benefits, and increased Medicare and Medicaid copayments have shifted greater financial responsibility for health care to the poor and elderly (Iglehart, 1982; Brown, 1983). Yet the structure, purpose and financing of the major health and social welfare programs themselves remains little changed (Glazer, 1984).

Nor has the welfare state's network of regulatory controls been dismantled. While the Reagan administration has slowed the growth of new regulatory initiatives, its deregulatory program is widely regarded as a failure (Green, 1983; Lublin, 1983; Pear, 1983). From nursing home standards to environmental protection, attempts at deregulation have generally encountered overwhelming political resistance. Federal funding has been largely withdrawn from the health planning program provided by Health Systems Agencies on the basis that health planning hinders competition, but many states have chosen to maintain these programs (*New York Times,* June 10, 1984, p. 1). Although the PSRO program was emasculated in the early 1980s and targeted by the Administration for elimination (Mihalski, 1984: 50–53), the legislation instituting a prospective rate-setting system for Medicare mandates the continuance of functions by Professional Review Organizations (PRO's). The purpose of PRO's is to insure that in response to strong incentives to eliminate "unnecessary" services, standards of quality do not fall below professional norms.

With the exception of one major addition, prospective rate-setting in the Medicare program, the regulatory landscape appears largely unaltered. It is no small irony that this, the most far-reaching health system reform achieved by this administration, is itself a form of regulation. Comprehensive reforms based on the market-competition model are backed by neither political consensus nor a particular constituency (Brown, 1983). Even among their own political allies, conservative backers of procompetitive reforms have found little support: neither insurance companies nor the medical profession supports policies to increase competition within the health care sector. After a brief flirtation with the concept of deregulation, health care providers appear to have quickly understood that they have little to gain from increased competition. As Reinhardt has noted, "a competitive market system is, after all, a social arrangement whereby life is made hell for providers to make life cheap and easy for consumers" (1982: 23). Competitive reforms appear to have found some success largely on the state level where innovations such as competitive bidding for Medicaid provider contracts and increased enrollment of Medicaid clients in HMO's have been used to complement, not to replace, cost-containment regulation (*New York Times*, Nov. 20, 1983, p. 30).

Although concerns about cost containment still dominate discussions of health care policy, government cutbacks in assistance to the poor have prompted renewed concern about access to care. Recently, proposals to extend federally provided health insurance benefits to the unemployed and medically indigent have received serious congressional consideration.

Within health care it appears that the swing to the right has run its course. The debate between competition and regulation, however, now appears muddled. The stability of health and welfare programs in the face of proposals for radical change is mirrored by—and perhaps grounded in—the stability of public attitudes toward these programs. Analyses of public opinion polls do not reveal a massive shift to the right in political ideology over the past decade: public support for the regulatory and entitlement programs that comprise the welfare state has remained surprisingly stable (Dowling, 1982; Ladd, 1983; Navarro, 1983; Robinson, 1984). Even that bellwether of liberalism, national health insurance, so decisively rejected by conservative leadership in Congress and the executive branch, appears to have retained approximately the same level of high public support (Ladd, 1983).

In the 1970s, NHI faded from the political agenda because it was felt that any national health insurance plan would only add to already uncontrollable health care expenditures. In the 1980s, it appears possible that costs may be the galvanizing issue in reestablishing momentum for the passage of a form of NHI with stringent cost controls (Schroeder, 1981). Such a plan is already garnering support both from industry, as a way to ease the burden of paying for health benefits for its workers,[2] and from hospitals and physicians as a way to guarantee payment in an increasingly competitive environment[3] (Ginzberg et al, 1981), just as they supported Blue Cross and Blue Shield in an earlier era (Somers and Somers, 1961). Increasing governmental responsibility for health care is one way to deal with difficult and necessary decisions about the limits to the society's overall allocation for health care. Certainly it is not lost on U.S. observers that the opportunity to create a national health care budget as in England, Canada, and many European countries offers certain advantages in the cost-containment struggle. For example, the continued popularity of the British National Health Service under the present conservative government is, in part, due to the fact that the NHS is regarded as the most effective way to ration health care (Klein, 1984).

Now, as in the past, a number of national health insurance proposals are at various stages of congressional scrutiny. At least in the immediate future none is given a serious chance of passage. The bills embody a wide range of approaches—from "catastrophic" coverage to those which would fundamentally reform the financing and delivery of health services. Whether the "health care cost crisis" will eventually provoke strong political support for an NHI proposal that would transcend the largely incremental proposals of the past is unclear. Undoubtedly, however, such a proposal would also encounter strong opposition from a range of powerful interest groups.

It is clear, however, that the questions confronting national health care policy, including the likely re-emergence of the NHI debate, offer many continuities with those of previous decades. Defining the appropriate role of a federal system of government in addressing key health systems goals is a persistent issue for analysis and debate.

Policy Implications of Physicians' Attitudes

A Framework

What is the relevance of physicians' attitudes for the design and implementation of health care policies? Although it is commonly believed that the medical profession is not as powerful as it was two decades ago, before the passage of Medicare, the views of physicians are still taken into account in decisions about health care. For example, the results of a recent survey of the attitudes of physicians toward various mechanisms of cost control, similar to issues we investigated in 1973, were considered important enough to be reported at a congressional hearing (Jeffe and Jeffe, 1984: 47). Many Washington observers still view the AMA as one of the most powerful lobbies in town. Its Political Action Committees spend millions of dollars annually ("Interest groups pressing for earlier, more active role in electoral process," 1983).

But to whom do policy-makers really listen—to pronouncements by leaders of organized medicine or to reports of the findings of attitude surveys of physicians, responding as individuals? To answer that question requires a sense of how the political process works. We see it as a system of competing interest groups, not as an atomized collection of individuals. This view emphasizes the political role of organized medicine. But this view does not imply that the preferences of individual members of the profession are irrelevant to the political process. We can point to both *direct* effects and, more substantially, to *indirect* effects.

Individual physicians can have direct effects if they influence individual decision-makers, one-to-one; and also if decision-makers are influenced by reports of systematic studies of physicians' attitudes toward health policies and programs. Surveys may set limits to the range of options considered by policy-makers; or they may be used to support or attack predetermined positions (see Meltsner, 1972; Colombotos, Kirchner and Millman, 1976).[4] Further, it has long been recognized that physicians' critical position in the health care system affects its operation. "It is impossible," says Fuchs (1974), "to make significant changes in the medical field without changing physician behavior" (Fuchs, 1974). To the extent that physicians' attitudes are linked to their practice behavior, they may spell the difference between success and failure in the implementation of health care programs.

The attitudes of physicians enter indirectly into the political process in two ways. First, leaders of organized medicine are influenced, or at least take into account, what they perceive to be the views of their constituents in developing policy positions.

Second, the influence of medical leaders is enhanced to the extent that they can claim that their positions represent the views of their constituents. But that claim may be challenged when individuals or segments of the profession speak out against official organizational policies. For example, when the government brought an antitrust suit against the AMA in 1938 for denying membership to physicians working for Group Health Association (GHA) under a prepayment system, the fact that several distinguished members of the AMA supported GHA brought into question whether the association could speak for its members in an authoritative fashion (Truman, 1971: 169–170).

Since systematic studies of physicians' attitudes may also support or challenge that claim, such studies become politically significant. The AMA opposed surveys of physicians on these grounds until the early seventies ("The Insider's Newsletter," 1965; Tatalovich, 1971: 198), when it began to sponsor its own.[5]

Physicians' Attitudes in the Mid-Eighties— and in the Decade Ahead

What are the current political and health care views of physicians—and how are they likely to change? For an answer we rely on projections from our own data in 1973, on more recent studies of physicians' attitudes, and on objective trends in the organization of health care that both reflect and influence the attitudes of doctors.

Our findings draw an ideological profile of the profession that will influence its thinking for some time; in a word, despite a politically conservative shift in recent years in the society at large (a shift, as we noted earlier, that is not as massive or as extensive as is commonly believed), the profession will be generally more liberal, especially with respect to changes in the organization of health care. This prediction is based on (1) ongoing changes in the social and professional characteristics of physicians, which are in turn related to their attitudes, and (2) generational differences between younger and older physicians in their attitudes.

Major changes in the composition of the profession include:

- a sharp increase in the proportion of women to a point where, if current medical school enrollment practices continue, within a few decades women will comprise a fifth of the nation's physicians;
- an increase in the proportion of salaried, group-based physicians;
- an increase in the proportion of physicians in primary care specialties and declines in specialties in which there are current or projected oversupplies, notably certain surgical specialties.

These changes indicate that the thinking of physicians will generally follow a more liberal trend.[6] Sharp attitudinal differences between broadly defined generations, specifically with respect to group practice, peer reviews, and task delegation, also suggest an increasingly liberal climate in the profession in relation to those aspects of medical practice.

Recent studies of physicians' attitudes show that group practice and peer reviews ("second opinion" programs and utilization reviews by third-party payers); a system incorporating nurse-practitioners, mid-wives, and physicians' assistants; capitation payment; and growth of the HMO concept were all acceptable to near majorities or comfortable majorities of physicians (Louis Harris and Associates, 1981, 1984; American Medical Association, 1983b). The identification of trends based on comparisons between these findings and our 1973 findings is risky because of differences in the wording of questions used in the studies. Our impression, however, taking these differences in the wording of questions into account, is that the current climate of physician opinion is more favorable toward these health care issues than it was a decade ago, a conclusion that was anticipated in generational differences we found in 1973.

But beyond attitude trends indicated and sustained by generational differences at a given point in time, objective changes in the health care environment (translate: "period effects") also indicate changes in the attitudes of physicians. Thus, for example, the growth of group and of salaried practice both *reflects* positive changes in the attitudes of physicians toward these arrangements, to the extent that physicians are free to choose among alternative forms of practice, it *influences* the attitudes of physicians, to the extent that experience in these settings has a socializing effect on their attitudes.

On some issues, however, physicians' support has declined since the mid-seventies; and on others, there is considerable resistance. The proportion of physicians who felt that there was "a need for national health insurance" dropped sharply from 53 percent in 1978 to 30 percent in 1982, as we indicated in Chapter 2 (56%, it will be recalled, were "in favor . . . of some form of national health insurance" in our 1973 study). The proportion among the general population remained both higher and stable (between 64 and 68%) during this period.

But NHI will re-emerge—within the decade, if not in the immediate future. Public support continues to be high and, according to some observers, may even rise as a result of fear of runaway medical expenses; the concern of big business about the upwardly spiralling cost of providing health care benefits for its employees is forcing some of its leaders to turn to NHI, with controls on cost, as a solution; and, finally, the medical profession may support NHI as a means for providing a floor on the income of physicians in the face of increasing competition caused by physician oversupply. Physicians may come to see NHI not only as inevitable, but as desirable. Physician support of some form of NHI is likely to be further facilitated by their earlier acceptance and positive experiences with Medicare. Physician support for alternative NHI plans, however, will vary depending on specific components of those plans.

The two proposals for containing the cost of health care that were least acceptable in the 1984 Harris poll cited earlier were: the DRG concept ("a system in which the fees paid to doctors and hospitals for treating all patients with particular diagnoses are fixed"), which was acceptable to only a third of the physicians; and "government price controls of doctors' and hospital fees," acceptable to only 13 percent.[7] The incorporation of these proposals into NHI is likely to be at the center of the debate about NHI alternatives. Whether or not they are a part of the NHI debate, however, these two related issues—the potential of DRG's for spawning explicit protocols and standards for care and the direct government regulation of physicians' fees—are the key issues impinging on the medical profession in the immediate future.[8] The one strikes at the clinical autonomy of physicians—their claim to exercise their individual discretionary judgment in a given case, unhampered by rules and regulations. The other strikes more directly at their pocketbook.

Physicians distinguish between different types of reviews (Chapter 2): they are less likely to accept reviews based on explicit standards and protocols, even by "peers," than informal reviews based on implicit standards. Explicit standards conjure up the spectre of "cookbook" medicine; informal reviews are associated with collegial consultation and advice (Goss, 1961).

In response to recent proposals mandating fixed fees for physicians under Medicare, the AMA proclaimed that many doctors would refuse to treat Medicare patients rather than accept a fixed-fee system; that such fee-schedules would be an unwarranted intrusion into the practice of medicine and a form of enslavement in medicine (*New York Times*, June 15, 1984, p. A-15). The rhetoric is strikingly similar to the AMA's response to Medicare two decades ago, just before it was passed, warning that doctors would refuse to treat Medicare patients (Chapter 6).

During the next decade clinical protocols and standards, spearheaded by the DRG concept, will probably exercise an increasing influence on the clinical decision-making of physicians. In addition, the fees of physicians will probably be fixed, first under Medicare, and then under other government-financed programs, such as NHI.

Physicians will adapt to both. Organized medicine is likely to be invited, if not required, to play a major role in the development and implementation of both programs: in the formulation of clinical protocols and in the negotiation of fee schedules, a role it plays in many countries with national health insurance systems. Moreover, organized medicine will seize the opportunity to be involved as a means of influencing the development of both, just as it has participated in Medicare, PSRO's, and other programs.

In an ironic turn of events, organized medicine may turn to the federal government, its traditional adversary, against for-profit chains providing medical care. The clinical autonomy of physicians—and their pocket-books—are likely to fare better if clinical protocols and physicians' fees are negotiated between government and organized medicine than if they are left to the whim of market forces, a market in which the for-profits chains would have the upper hand over individual physicians competing with each other.[9] Collective autonomy would replace individual auton-omy in both clinical decision-making and in physician reimbursement.

One unknown in this scenario is which segments of organized medi-cine will gain control of these functions: Will it be the American Medical Association or the specialty societies? Our research points to the great diversity of physicians' opinion. We identified pockets of relative support and opposition within the profession to major political and health care issues. Some of these lines of division—worksetting, specialty, geogra-phy—identify special constituencies of physicians represented by special organizations. In the face of these divisions, the AMA is hard-pressed to justify its claim as spokesman and bargaining agent for the entire profes-sion.

Our findings, which indicate a general congruence between the atti-tudes of leaders and members of the AMA and its constituent state and county medical societies (Chapter 7), strengthen the claim that the AMA and its constituent bodies speak for the profession as a whole. That claim is weakened, however, by the growing number of physicians who join neither the county and state medical societies nor the AMA, and who, it will be recalled, are more liberal than leaders and members. The leader-ship of the AMA and its state and county medical societies thus may speak in the future for a progressively shrinking segment of the profes-sion. With the expanding number of "nonmembers" and their represen-tation, potentially, by other organizations, the power of the AMA will be further challenged.[10] To the extent that the AMA is unable to contain the diverging interests of various segments of the profession, organized medi-cine as a whole will be further fragmented and weakened.

Notes

1. For an analysis of recent changes in health care within such a historical context, see Stevens (1984).

2. Members of the board of the Chrysler Corporation, including Lee A. Iacocca, its chairman, and Joseph A. Califano, Jr., who was Secretary of Health, Education and Welfare, under Carter, have expressed support for NHI (*New York Times*, March 5, 1984, p. A1).

3. The proportion of physicians who thought that there were "too many" doctors in their community rose from 33 percent in 1981 to 45 percent in 1983; and the proportions were higher among younger physicians (American Medical Association, 1983b: 4–5). Also a third of the physicians interviewed in 1983 reported that the number of their uncollected bills had increased over the previous year (American Medical Association, 1983b: 8).

4. To demonstrate "a grassroots physicians' support for the PSRO concept," Senator Wallace Bennett, sponsor of the PSRO bill, introduced into the Congressional Record (July 11, 1974) a news release reporting on physicians' favorable attitudes toward peer reviews in our 1973 national study (see Colombotos, Kirchner, and Millman, 1976.)

5. In a different context, Solomon Barkin, Research Director of the Textile Workers Union of America, objected to the partisan use of surveys of labor by management: "the union [leadership] is clubbed through all channels of communication with the results of supposedly objective surveys of worker opinion, and *its position and right to speak for its members strongly challenged*" (*emphasis added*; quoted in Hyman, 1955: 49).

6. These projections must, of course, be qualified by the possibility that the direction and strength of the relationship between certain social and professional characteristics and certain attitudes can change historically. It has been argued, for example, that voting habits and political views became more strongly associated with socioeconomic status during and after the Depression of the 1930s than before (Berelson et al., 1954: 59–61, 91; Campbell et al., 1960: 356–360; Abramson, 1975; note also the emerging "gender gap" in American politics). Finally, our data show that, whereas among the senior physicians, general and family practitioners were among the most conservative on health care issues, among medical students, those choosing general and family practice were among the most liberal. Also, changes in the composition of the profession, for example, the increasing proportion of women, may itself affect the relationship between physicians' gender and their attitudes. (For a discussion of the effects of "relative numbers" of women physicians on the socialization of both genders, see Shapiro and Jones, 1979: 237–245).

Our findings establishing the influence of both early and later sources of socialization on physicians' attitudes bear directly on the pragmatic question of the relative importance of medical school admissions criteria, professional training, and professional worksettings for attitudes and behavior of physicians. If the objective is to promote certain attitudes and behavior in physicians, say the acceptance of salaried practice or sensitivity to psychosocial aspects of patient care, it would be useful to know if relevant attitudes are formed *before* medical training and vary according to identifiable social background characteristics (e.g., gender, ethnicity, socioeconomic background) or whether they are formed *during* medical training or, even *later*, in medical practice, and vary according to types of medical training and practice settings.

The answer would suggest whether changes could then be instituted in admissions criteria, professional training, or professional worksettings to achieve the desired objective. Up to recently, health care issues have received scant attention in medical school. But with the growth of educational programs dealing with ethical issues, health care costs, and related matters in health care delivery, professional training may influence the attitudes of physicians toward these issues more strongly than in the past.

7. It is difficult to reconcile the finding that "government price controls of doctors' and hospital fees" were acceptable to only 13 percent of physicians (in 1984) with our finding

that "a plan (under NHI) under which all doctors would be paid a *fixed fee* for each service, negotiated by a committee on which physicians are represented" was "agreeable" to *61 percent* (in 1973). We suspect that the provision in the latter question that the fees be "negotiated by a committee on which physicians are represented" made the plan more acceptable to physicians than it would have been otherwise.

8. The DRG program covering charges for inpatient care under Medicare went into effect in the fall of 1983. A year later, Congress imposed a 15-month freeze on physicians' fees for Medicare patients. The same bill provided for a study to investigate the feasibility of national fee schedules for physicians.

9. One may speculate about the implications of the growth of for-profit medicine for the health care views of physicians and ultimately for their medical practice behavior. To what extent and in what ways will the more open expression of naked, direct economic self-interest edge out professional norms and values, such as the service ethic and trust, which mute (some would say "mask") their self-serving interests, as the rationale underpinning the attitudes and behavior of physicians? And how will these developments impact on traditional views that distinguish medicine as a profession from medicine as a business (see Relman, 1980; Gray, 1983; Luft, 1983; and Veatch, 1983)?

10. For example, note the following challenge in a statement issued by the progressive Physicians' Forum:

> We see the need for a new organization devoted to the protection and advancement of salaried physicians. The AMA and its local groupings, traditional voices of medicine, are historically locked into representing the anachronistic cottage-industry physician (1982: 5)

Appendix

In this Appendix we describe the sampling designs, methods of data collection, and measures and scales used in the 1973 national study. The sampling design and the methods of data collection used in the New York State longitudinal study are described in Chapters 1 and 6.

Sampling Designs

Following is a brief description of the sampling design for each group in the national study (see Table A-1).

SENIOR PHYSICIANS. This is a national probability sample of all active physicians, excluding interns and residents, in the AMA physician file on December 31, 1972. The universe was stratified by major activity (office-based and hospital-based practice, medical teaching, administration, and research) and state. Physicians in office-based practice were sampled at a rate of 0.9 percent, and all others at the rate of 3 percent.

INTERNS AND RESIDENTS (HOUSESTAFF). The sampling design provides a national probability sample of interns and residents drawn from the AMA file in the Fall, 1972, based on records provided by all hospitals with approved training programs. The sample was stratified by state.

MEDICAL STUDENTS. The sampling of medical students was designed both to permit a contextual analysis of students from different types of medical schools and to provide a nationally representative sample. A two-

Table A-1. Sampling Plan and Field Results

	Total universe	Sampling rate (%)	Sample size	No. of respondents	Net response rate[a] (%)
Senior physicians					
Patient care					
Office-based practice	196,919	0.9	1,767	1,306	75
Hospital-based practice	34,761	3.0	1,042	779	77
Other professional activity:					
Medical teaching	5,804	3.0	175	140	81
Administration	11,263	3.0	337	269	82
Research	10,093	3.0	302	219	75
Total Senior physicians	258,840[b]	—	3,623	2,713	75
Interns & Residents	57,457[b]	3.0	1,721	1,303	76
Medical students	46,353[c]	—	4,125	3,414	84
Special samples:					
(Prepaid group practice)[d]					
PGP 1	297	—	200	155	78
PGP 2	850	—	200	152	77
Medical faculty[e]	2,008	40.0	803	576	72

[a]Net response rate is calculated on the "eligible" sample, i.e., after eliminating doctors who had died, retired, or moved out of the country (or students who were no longer in the sampled school) between sample selection and field work. It includes in the base those who refused to participate in the study, those who could not be located, and those who were temporarily ill or otherwise unavailable.

[b]The universe for "senior physicians" and interns and residents is the total number of "active" physicians in the AMA physician file as of December 31, 1972. This cut-off date is used by the AMA for their annual report of national statistics. Our definition includes both federal and nonfederal physicians in the 50 states.

[c]"Medical education in the United States, 1972–73," 1973: 902.

[d]The universe for physicians in each of two large prepaid group practices includes full-time physicians in early 1973. In PGP 2, one of 14 clinics in the group was excluded because it would not cooperate. A sample size, rather than sampling rate, was set in advance for each group.

[e]The universe for Medical Faculty includes all full-time physician faculty in the roster maintained by the Association of American Medical Colleges (AAMC) for the academic year 1971–72 in a subsample of 11 of the 24 medical schools sampled for medical students. The national universe of full-time medical faculty in 1971–72 was 18,415.

Sampling weights: In order to adjust for the different sampling rates among senior physicians and not to inflate the totals, office-based practitioners were assigned a weight of 1.566 and all others, .476.

step procedure sampled, first, schools, and then students within those schools.

From an analysis of the correlations of various characteristics of medical schools based on data provided by the Association of American Medical Colleges (AAMC) and on other sources, 24 schools were selected within the key strata defined by geographic region (four Census regions) and public versus private auspices. A one-third sample of students was drawn from each of the four classes in the twenty-four schools selected proportional to size from the universe of all four year medical schools which had granted the M.D. degree in June, 1972, and had students enrolled in each class in 1972–73 (excluding a few "developing schools").

SPECIAL SAMPLE OF MEDICAL FACULTY. Our original objective was to select a sample of medical faculty from the same schools from which students were selected for a comparative analysis of faculty and students—a sample that would also be nationally representative of physicians in "medical teaching" as a component of a national sample of senior physicians.

This was not possible because the medical faculty roster maintained by the Association of American Medical Colleges (AAMC) did not correspond to the AMA's "medical teaching" category. We therefore sampled instead AAMC-defined faculty from a random one-half of the medical schools for student-faculty comparisons and selected a regular sample from the AMA's "medical teaching" category to complete the national representation of "senior physicians" in all activities.

SPECIAL SAMPLES OF PHYSICIANS IN TWO PREPAID GROUP PRACTICE PLANS. Samples of 200 full-time physicians in each of two large prepaid group plans—one on the East Coast (with 297 full-time physicians) and the other on the West Coast (with 850 full-time physicians)—were selected for special analysis and comparison with physicians in solo, fee-for-service practice.

A Note on Statistical Significance Tests

The appropriateness of tests of statistical significance in survey research has been a topic of controversy over the years (see Lipset, Trow, and Coleman, 1956: 427–432; Merton, Reader, and Kendall, 1957: 301–5; and Selvin, 1957).

The use of such tests is even more problematic in our analysis because both the New York State longitudinal sample and the 1973 national sample of senior physicians were weighted. Since most commonly used

significance tests assume simple random sampling, they are not legitimate, in a strict statistical sense, in weighted samples (Blalock, 1979: 566–7).

Nevertheless, bearing these caveats in mind, we computed conventional test statistics for selected tables to guide our data analysis. The
significance levels of these test statistics are not to be interpreted literally
as probabilities of type I error (Blalock, 1979: 109–112). It should also be
noted that because of the relatively large samples, some relationships,
though significant at the .01 level, are not particularly "strong" by
conventional survey analysis standards.

Data Collection Procedures

Two pretests were conducted. In the first, telephone interviews were
concluded with 33 medical students, 24 housestaff members, and 101
senior physicians in June, 1972, by National Opinion Research Center
(NORC) and project staff. The second pretest included an experimental
comparison of the mail and telephone methods among 504 medical
students and housestaff members and telephone interviews with 188
senior physicians between November, 1972, and January, 1973.

Experimental Comparisons Between Personal, Telephone, and Mail Methods

Early studies generally showed that personal, face-to-face interviews were
more likely to elicit socially acceptable responses than self-administered
questionnaires because of the "social component of involvement" between interviewer and respondent (Hyman, 1954: 138–139). The telephone interview falls between the personal interview and the self-administered questionnaire in the opportunity for such involvement. In an
experimental comparison of the telephone and personal interview methods among a subsample of respondents in the first wave of the New York
State longitudinal study, however, we found essentially no differences in
the proportions giving socially acceptable responses according to the two
methods (Colombotos, 1969a).

In the national study, the original plan called for data from physicians,
including interns and residents, to be obtained by telephone interview,
and from medical students by mail questionnaire. Since a major objective
of the study was to compare the attitudes of medical students, housestaff,
and senior physicians, it was critical to determine if responses were
affected by the methods by which they were obtained. Accordingly, in-

cluded in the second pretest was an experimental comparison between the mail questionnaire and the telephone interview method among interns and residents in 15 hospitals and medical students in two medical schools not in the national sample of 24 medical schools. Interns and residents were included in the experiment both to test the feasibility of using the less expensive mail questionnaire among them and to extend the generalizability of the experimental comparison of responses obtained by the two methods.

Prior to analysis of the experimental data, three of the Columbia University project staff acted independently as "judges," rating all questionnaire items according to whether they had a high, medium, or low component of social desirability. For example, we agreed doctors would perceive greater social approval for a response that they "view patients as individuals" rather than as "examples of disease entities" (Q. 58) and that desire for money and prestige played no part in their choice of medicine as a career (Q. 54). In addition, we assumed that the lay public, as represented by the interviewer, would be seen as more approving of doctors who gave "liberal" rather than "conservative" responses on economic and health care delivery issues.

The three judges agreed on 18 items as being "high" in social desirability and also agreed on the "desirable" response category. This permitted us to make 36 comparisons of method by using the same 18 items for medical students and, separately, for housestaff members.

Only two items showed a difference according to method of ten or more percentage points in the predicted direction for both groups. One of these, an open-ended question on the main problem facing the medical profession, was dropped from the main study. The other item was "expected income at peak of career." Our prediction was that income expectations would be lower when given by phone than by mail. (The difference was minimized when the seven response categories were trichotomized.)

We concluded that the mail and telephone methods yielded sufficiently comparable results; more precisely, that the potential problem of social desirability did not apply to the types of questions, target population, and interviewing styles in this study.

Field Procedures

The field operations for the final study samples began on February 24, 1973, for interns and residents, when mail questionnaires were sent out; on February 22 for senior physicians, when the first of eight regional briefing sessions for approximately 100 National Opinion Research Center interviewers and their immediate supervisors was held (a senior NORC staff member and a Columbia University project staff member led each of these sessions); and on April 6 for medical students, when the first group of mail questionnaires were sent out.

The bulk of interviews and questionnaires were completed by the end of May, with the exception of about 700 mail questionnaires and telephone interviews from medical students obtained in June, and a few dozen in July.

With only a few exceptions, a net response rate (i.e., after eliminating from the base "sampling losses," such as those physicians who were deceased or retired or who had left the country and students and faculty no longer in the sampled school), a net response rate of at least 75 percent was obtained in each of the 37 cells representing major activity and housestaff status in each of the four major geographic regions (24 cells), medical school faculty (11 cells), and each of the two prepaid group practice plans (2 cells); and in each of the 96 (4 × 24) cells representing each class and medical school.

Although a combination of the telephone interview and the mail questionnaire was used for each of the three major respondent groups, the first and main approach varied in number for each group. All medical students and housestaff members were initially mailed questionnaires, and all senior physicians were initially assigned to telephone interviews, except for mail questionnaires to 24 doctors in Alaska and Hawaii (only 6 of the 24 responded). Nonrespondents, after several contacts by the original method, were offered the alternative method. Ultimately, 96 percent of the senior physician respondents in the national sample were interviewed by phone, as were 13 percent of housestaff members and 8 percent of students.

Senior Physicians

The first contact with individuals in the senior physician sample was a letter over the signature of John H. Bryant, M.D., then Director of the Columbia University School of Public Health, giving a brief description of the study and asking for the respondent's cooperation. This was followed by a telephone call from an interviewer to make an appointment to do the interview.

Intensive follow-up procedures included: repeated telephone calls if a physician did not respond to the initial letter; a second and third letter requesting cooperation and reassignment to another interviewer if the physician or his or her receptionist refused to make an appointment during an initial contact; inquiries of state medical societies, state boards of medical licensure, the armed forces, the Educational Council for Foreign Medical Graduates, and other organizations to check addresses and telephone numbers of physicians who could not be contacted; a self-administered questionnaire mailed to the physician for completion if that form was preferred in place of an interview.

Interns and Residents

A series of three mailings to interns and residents on February 24, March 12, and March 30, with covering letters from Dr. Bryant, yielded responses from 49 percent of the original sample. A telephone followup of the nonrespondents, beginning April 19, produced another 16 percent from mail questionnaires and 12 percent from telephone interviews, most of them by the end of May.

Followup activities included inquiries at hospitals, the Educational Council for Foreign Medical Graduates, and other sources to check addresses and telephone numbers of respondents who could not be contacted.

Medical Students

Two mailings to medical students with covering letters from Dr. Bryant—a first mailing during a 10-day interval beginning April 6, and a second mailing beginning April 25—yielded returns from 66 percent of the original sample by May 21.

In 18 of the 24 medical schools, questionnaires were mailed directly to the students at their local addresses; in three institutions, questionnaires were mailed to the students in care of the school and distributed in their school mail boxes; and in three other schools, which did not release their students' local addresses, stamped questionnaires with students' names were sent to the school and local addresses were added by the Dean's office and mailed out.

In the middle of May we considered sending a third mailing to the nonrespondents, but because the semester was coming to a close for a large number of classes in the schools, we were concerned about losing contact with students, especially the graduating seniors. We chose instead to assign the nonrespondents for immediate telephone followup beginning May 21.[1] We received an additional 421 mail questionnaires (10% of the sample) and completed 296 telephone interviews (7% of the sample) after this date.

Testing for Nonresponse Bias

In comparing respondents and nonrespondents among senior physicians and housestaff members on background characteristics available from the AMA, no difference as large as 10 percent in any one category was found, although some smaller differences were statistically significant at the .01 level (using X^2 or Yates corrected X^2 where applicable). Among senior physicians, nonrespondents were slightly older, less likely to be board-certified, and in the "radiology, anesthesiology, or pathology" specialty category, and more likely to be foreign medical graduates and to be in the midatlantic states. Among housestaffs, nonrespondents also were older and slightly more likely to be board-certified; there were no significant differences by country of graduation.

Measures and Scales

In most cases in this section, we have included the question, exactly as worded in the interview, on which a measure is based. In a few cases we have indicated only the question number. All questions appear in an exact reproduction of the Interview Schedule immediately following this section.

Where we have conceived of responses as constituting an ordinal scale (none, except possibly age and income, constitutes an interval scale), we have included the value assigned to each response in parentheses following that response. These values were used in computing total scale scores and in calculating statistics.

Unless indicated otherwise, scale scores were computed as follows: total scores were divided by the number of items answered to yield scores in the range 1–5. Respondents who answered fewer than half the items were excluded. For cross-tabulation analysis, scores were collapsed into five categories with cutting points as close as possible to quintiles among senior physicians. Percent "liberal" or "favor" in Tables 4-1, 4-2, 5-1, and 7-1 are those in types "1" and "2," the most liberal 30 to 40 percent of the overall distribution.

The internal consistency of items in attitude scales was tested by Cronbach's "alpha" (Nunnally, 1967: 195), based on the responses of senior physicians. The alphas for housestaff and medical students were remarkably similar to those for senior physicians.

Unidimensionality was tested by factor analysis (varimax rotation, using "PA2" in the SPSS manual—see Nie et al., 1975: 474–476, 480). Each scale that was retained produced only one factor, using a minimum eigenvalue of 1.

Socioeconomic Background (SEB)

A socioeconomic background (SEB) score was based on the respondent's father's education and the respondent's perceived social class background, as follows (see note 2 in Chapter 3):

> Q. 84. What was the last grade or year in school your father completed?
> Eighth grade or less (1)
> Some high school (2)
> High school graduate (3)
> Business or technical school after high school (4)
> Some college (5)
> College graduate (6)
> More than college (7)

> Q. 92. Which one of the following comes closest to describing the social class your parents belonged to when you were in your teens . . .
> upper class (10), or
> upper middle class (8), or
> lower middle class (6), or
> working class (4), or
> lower class (2)?

Thus, scores ranged from 3 (lowest socioeconomic background) to 17 (highest).

In the cross-tabulation analysis, physicians whose fathers were physicians were identified separately and the scores of the remainder were collapsed into four categories, as indicated in Table 4-1. In the hierarchical multiple regression, physician-fathers were not identified separately and the raw SEB score was used.

Religious Background

> Q. 81. In what religion were you brought up?
> Protestant
> Roman Catholic

Jewish
Other (Specify)
None

Generation-in-the-United States

Based on responses to Q.'s 78 and 79, and classified as follows:

Respondent was born outside the United States (first-generation) (1)
Respondent was born in the United States and one or both parents were born outside the United States (second-generation) (2)
Respondent was born in the United States and both parents were born in the United States (third-or-more generation) (3)

Degree of Urbanization

Based on the U.S. Census classification of ZIP code of physician's mailing address, as follows:

Up to population of 10,000 (1)
10,000 to 25,000 (2)
25,000 to 50,000 (3)
Non-metropolitan, 50,000 or over (4)
Potential Standard Metropolitan Statistical Area (SMSA) (5)
SMSA, 50,000 to 500,000 (6)
SMSA, 500,000 to 1 million (7)
SMSA, 1 to 5 million (8)
SMSA, 5 million or over (9)

In the cross-tabulation analysis, these nine categories were collapsed into three categories as follows: categories 1-4, 5-7, 8-9 (see Table 4-1).

Medical Specialty

Based on responses to Q.'s 1 and 1A, and classified as follows:

General/family practice
Surgical specialties—include general, neurological, thoracic, plastic, and orthopedic surgery; obstetrics and gynecology, ophthalmology, otolaryngology, urology
Medical specialties—include internal medicine, pediatrics, cardiology, dermatology, neurology, pulmonary diseases

Psychiatry
All others—include anesthesiology, pathology, radiology, occupational medicine, public health, and "others"

Worksetting

A typology was constructed based on *main activity* (whether most hours were spent in teaching, patient care, research, or administration, based on responses to Q's. 2, 3, 7, and 8); *organization of work* (Q. 4A); and main *method of reimbursement* (Q's. 4 and 95B). Types were classified as follows:

Patient care
   Individual or partnership with one other physician,
       fee-for-service (1);
   Group or hospital-based, fee-for-service (2);
   Group or hospital-based, salaried (3);
Nonpatient care (teaching, research, administration) (4)

Board Certification

Based on the AMA's Physician Master File.

Professional Income

95. A. In which of these following groups was your net professional income in 1972, that is, after expenses, but before taxes. Just these broad groups . . .
   Under $20,000 (1)
   $20,000 to $29,999 (2)
   $30,000 to $39,999 (3)
   $40,000 to $49,999 (4)
   $50,000 to $59,999 (5)
   $60,000 to $79,999 (6)
   $80,000 or more? (7)

B. About what percent of this was salary?
   None
   1–24%
   25–49%
   50–74%
   75–99%
   100%

Father's Political Identification

Q. 87. In his political thinking would you describe your father as . . .
radical left (1), or
liberal (2), or
middle-of-the-road (3), or
conservative (4), or
radical right (5)?

Father's Political Party Preference

Q. 86. Did your father consider himself a . . .
Democrat (1), or
Republican (5), or
some other party? (Specify)
Father never lived in the United States or not a citizen of the United
States

Career Values in Decision to Go into Medicine

Q. 54A. In your decision to go into medicine, how important was each of
the following . . .
very important (1)
somewhat important (3)
not at all important (5)?

Emphasis on Money

"Making a lot of money"

Emphasis on Autonomy

"Freedom from supervision in your work"

Respondent's Political Party Preference in Medical School

Q. 89. When you started medical school, did you consider yourself . . .
(If Independent) A. Did you identify more closely with the Democratic
or Republican party?
Strong Democrat (1.0)

Not very strong Democrat (1.66)
Independent—identified more closely with Democratic party (2.32)
Independent (2.98)
Independent—identified more closely with Republican party (3.64)
Not very strong Republican (4.30)
Strong Republican (5.00)

General Professional Satisfaction (alpha = 0.52)

Q. 52B. How about at the present time—do you have any doubts that medicine is the right profession for you—would you say you have . . .
serious doubts (5), or
slight doubts (3), or
no doubts at all (1)?

Q. 97. In general, how happy are you with your present career within medicine—are you . . .
very happy (1), or
somewhat happy (3), or
not happy (5)?

Scores ranged from most satisfied (2) to least satisfied (10).

Satisfaction with Professional Income

Q. 96. How satisfied are you with your professional income—are you . . .
very satisfied (1), or
somewhat satisfied (3), or
not satisfied (5)?

Economic-Welfare Liberalism Scale (alpha = 0.73)

Q. 34H. It is the responsibility of society, through its government to guarantee full employment.

Q. 34I. The government should play a bigger part in the economic life of the nation in order to distribute income more equally.

Q. 34J. Poverty could almost be done away with if we made certain basic changes in our social and economic system.

Q. 34K. The United States needs a complete restructuring of its basic institutions.

Responses were scored as follows: Agree strongly = 1, agree some-what = 2, disagree somewhat = 4, disagree strongly = 5.

Respondent's Political Identification

Q. 90. In your political thinking, do you consider yourself as . . .
  radical left (1), or
  liberal (2), or
  middle-of-the-road (3), or
  conservative (4), or
  radical right (5)?

Respondent's Present Political Party Preference

Q. 88. Do you consider yourself . . .
(If Independent) A. Do you identify more closely with the Democratic party or Republican party?
  Strong Democrat (1.0)
  Not very strong Democrat (1.66)
  Independent—identify more closely with Democratic party (2.32)
  Independent (2.98)
  Independent—identify more closely with Republican party (3.64)
  Not very strong Republican (4.30)
  Strong Republican (5.00)

Political Ideology Super-Scale (alpha = 0.78)

This scale was computed by adding the scores on the economic-welfare liberalism scale, political identification, and political party preference.
  Scores ranged from 15 (most liberal) to 3 (most conservative).

Government-in-Health Scale (alpha = 0.71)

Q. 20. Do you think the federal government should be involved a great deal, a fair amount, very little, or not at all, in decisions about each of the following:
  A. The construction of hospitals
  B. Medical school curricula

    C. Priorities in biomedical research
    D. Where doctors practice, by giving scholarships
    E. Students' choice of specialty, by giving scholarships
    F. Regulating the prescription drug industry.

Responses were scored as follows: A great deal = 1, a fair amount = 2, very little = 4, not at all = 5.

Government-in-Medicine (alpha = 0.62)

Q. 12. What is your opinion about Medicare—which pays for hospital and medical care for those 65 or over—are you personally . . .
    strongly in favor (1), or
    somewhat in favor (2), or
    somewhat opposed (4), or
    strongly opposed (5)?

Q. 20G. Do you think the federal government should be involved a great deal (1), a fair amount (2), very little (4), or not at all (5) in decisions about each of the following . . .
    Providing medical care to poor people

Q. 34B. It is the responsibility of society, through its government, to provide everyone with the best available medical care, whether he can afford it or not (strongly agree = 1, agree somewhat = 2, disagree somewhat = 4, disagree strongly = 5).

National Health Insurance Scale (alpha = 0.79)

Based on responses to the following questions:

Q. 22. Opinion of some form of NHI.

Q. 24. Preference for plan administered by private insurance versus federal government agency.

Q. 25. Preference for plan financed by tax-credit incentive for private insurance versus employer-employee contributions like Social Security.

Q. 27. Preference for plan that supports development of prepaid group practice versus one that does not.

Q. 31A, B. Assuming a compromise plan, expectations about extent of positive or negative effect on your work.

Q. 31C. Assuming a compromise plan, expectations about effect on quality of care.

Q. 31D. Assuming a compromise plan, expectations about long-run effect on unnecessary hospitalization.

Q. 31E. Assuming a compromise plan, expectations about long-run effect on unnecessary use of doctors' services.

Q. 31G. Assuming a compromise plan, would the federal government affect the professional freedom of the individual doctor?

Group Practice Scale (alpha = 0.81)

Q. 35A. Considering the following list of arrangements for practicing medicine, which one, in your opinion, is likely to lead to the *best medical care?*
Solo practice (1.0)
Partnership of two physicians (1.8)
A *small* group of 3 to 5 physicians, in *one* specialty (2.6)
A *small*, multi-specialty group (3.4)
A *large* group of 20 physicians or more *not* in a hospital (4.2)
A *large* group *based* in a hospital (5.0)

Q. 35B. Considering the same list of arrangements—suppose your income in all of these were the same—which one would you consider *most desirable* for yourself?

Q. 35C. And which one would be *least desirable* for yourself? (Scoring was reversed for this question.)

Peer Reviews Scale (alpha = 0.72)

Q. 39. More and more reviews are being made of doctors' work in *hospitals* by other doctors. What is your opinion of such a trend? (Strongly favor = 1, somewhat in favor = 2, somewhat opposed = 4, strongly opposed = 5.)

Q. 40. Now, how about reviews of doctors' work in their *offices* by other doctors. (Same codes as in Q. 39.)

Q. 26. Would you prefer a plan [under National Health Insurance] under which the work of doctors is routinely reviewed by a panel of practicing doctors, or a plan without such a system of reviews? (Prefer reviews strongly = 1, prefer reviews not strongly = 2, prefer no reviews not strongly = 4, prefer no reviews strongly = 5.)

Delegation of Tasks Scale (alpha = 0.85)

Q. 37. The use of nurse-practitioners and physicians' assistants has been proposed as one way to make better use of doctors' time. For each of the following duties, please tell me whether you think it is appropriate or not for such persons, assuming that they are properly trained and working under the supervision of a physician. (Appropriate = 1, not appropriate = 5.)

    1. Taking preliminary histories.
    2. Performing routine physical examinations.
    3. Differentiating between functional and organic murmurs.
    4. Deciding if suturing is necessary.
    5. Treating superficial corneal abrasions.
    6. Deciding whether a patient with what appears to be a minor complaint should be seen by a doctor.
    7. Deciding what allergy tests to do.
    8. Doing allergy tests.
    9. Diagnosing throat conditions.
    10. Deciding whether to prescribe an antibiotic for a sore throat.
    11. Prescribing medication for minor pain relief.
    12. Reading simple chest X-rays in a screening program.
    13. Doing minor suturing.
    14. Counselling a diabetic patient about his diet.
    15. Doing routine physical examinations on cardiac patients in follow-ups.
    16. Doing routine well-baby follow-ups.
    17. Doing routine pre-natal check-ups on the mother.
    18. Performing uncomplicated deliveries *in the hospital*.

Physician Reimbursement

Q. 28. Next—a question about how doctors should be paid under national health insurance. Would you be agreeable or not agreeable to . . .

    A. a plan under which all doctors are paid an *annual salary*?
    B. a plan under which family doctors would be paid an *annual amount* for each patient they take care of?
    C. a plan under which all doctors would be paid a *fixed fee* for each service, negotiated by a committee on which physicians are represented?
    D. a plan under which all doctors would be paid their own *customary fees* for each service?

Four types were constructed based on their responses to Q's 28A–D and scores assigned, as follows:

Agreeable to salary, regardless of responses to other three questions (1)

Agreeable to annual amount, but not to salary, regardless of responses to other two questions (2)

Agreeable to fixed fees, but not to salary or capitation, regardless of response to other question (3)

Agreeable to customary fees, but not to any of the other three methods (4).

Prepayment

Q. 36. Assuming that the physician gets paid a fee for each service, which of the following systems do you prefer . . .

one of *simple prepayment*, that is, which provides complete care to a family for a flat sum in advance

strongly (1.0)

not so strongly (1.5), or

one of *modified prepayment* where the patient must pay a *small fee*— say a dollar or two—for each service

strongly (2.0)

not so strongly (2.5), or

one in which the patient pays for each service and is *completely reimbursed* by a third party

not so strongly (3.5)

strongly (4.0), or

one in which the patient pays the whole fee for each service *without being reimbursed?*

not so strongly (4.5)

strongly (5.0)

(Q. 36A. How strongly do you feel about this . . . strongly, or not so strongly?)

Notes

1. Since two of the three schools that did not release their students' local addresses also did not release their students' telephone numbers, a third mailing was sent to these nonrespondents instead. In another school in which neither the Dean's office nor a student representative would release their graduating seniors' telephone numbers, we were able to obtain the names and addresses of the hospitals in which they would be interning from the Internship Matching Program for followup after July 1.

Interview Schedule

NATIONAL OPINION RESEARCH CENTER

University of Chicago

<u>PHYSICIANS VIEW SOCIAL CHANGE
IN MEDICINE</u>   <u>BEGIN DECK 40</u>

Physician's Name:_____   Case #_____
                                                            1-5/

1. Is your work concentrated in one of the specialties, or not?

                                    Yes (ASK A) 1   8/
                                    No, more than one
                                       specialty (ASK A) 2
                                    No, General Practice 3

    A. What is your primary specialty?

    Anesthesiology 01   Psychiatry 13   9-10/
    Cardiovascular diseases 02   Public Health 14
    Dermatology 03   Pulmonary diseases 15
    Family Practice 04   Radiology 16
    Internal Medicine 05   Surgery, general 17
    Neurology 06   Surgery, neurological 18
    Obstetrics & Gynecology 07   Surgery, thoracic 19
    Occupational medicine. 08   Surgery, plastic 20
    Ophthalmology 09   Surgery, orthopedic 21
    Otolaryngology (ENT) 10   Urology 22
    Pathology 11   Other (SPECIFY) 23
    Pediatrics 12
                                                 _____

like to ask how you spend your professional time--
be asking about teaching, patient care,
earch and administration.

Thinking of a recent typical work week, about
how many hours do you spend in teaching?

#_____   11-12/

None. 00

98 or more. 98

About how many hours do you spend in a typical
work week in all aspects of patient care (not
including time with patients seen in your
teaching or research)?

#_____   13-14/

None. 00

98 or more. 98

IF LESS THAN 10 HOURS, SKIP TO Q. 7

Is most of your practice...

fee-for-service, or (ASK A & B) . . 1   15/

salaried, or (ASK C) 2

share of group income, or (ASK C) . 3

some other arrangement? 4
(SPECIFY AND ASK C)

_____

IF "FEE-FOR-SERVICE", ASK A & B

A. Is that...

a solo practice, or 1   16/

a partnership with one other
physician, or 2

a small group of 3 to 5 physicians,
or 3

a larger group? (About how many?). 4

#_____   17-19/

B. Do you see most patients on...

referral from other doctors, or . . 1   20/

on self-referral? 2

IF "SALARIED", "SHARE OF GROUP INCOME", OR "OTHER",
ASK C

C. In what type of organization or group is that?

Non-government hospital 1   21/

Government hospital . . . . . ,. . . 2

Government agency other than
hospital (SPECIFY). 3

_____

Private industry 4

Prepaid group 5

Other (SPECIFY) _____ 6

IF "FEE-FOR-SERVICE" IN "GROUP", ASK Q. 5

5. A. Is the group...

a single specialty, or . 1   22/

multispecialty group?. . 2

B. About what proportion of the patients does
the group see on a prepaid basis...

all, or. 1   23/

more than half, or . . . 2

about half, or 3

less than half, or . . . 4

none?. 5

DON'T KNOW. 6

ASK EVERYONE IN PATIENT CARE

6. Is your office located...

in a hospital, or. . . . 1   24/

next to a hospital, or . 2

in some other place? . . 3

ASK EVERYONE

7. About how many hours a week do you spend
in research?

#_____   25-26

None 00

98 or more 98

IF 10 OR MORE HOURS, ASK A & B

A. Are you primarily in...

laboratory research, or. 1   27/

clinical research, or. . 2

both equally?. 3

B. In what type of organization do you
do research? Any others?

CODE AS MANY AS APPLY

Medical school 1   28/

Non-government hospital. 1   29/

Government hospital. . . 1   30/

Government agency other
than hospital (SPECIFY . 1   31/

_____

Private industry 1   32/

Other (SPECIFY). 1   33/

_____

8. In a typical work week, about how many hours do you spend as an administrator in an organization?

	# _____	34-35/
None	00	
98 or more	98	

IF 10 OR MORE HOURS, ASK A-C

A. In what type of organization are you an administrator?   Any others?

   CODE AS MANY AS APPLY

Medical school 1	36/
Non-government hospital 1	37/
Government hospital 1	38/
Government agency other than hospital (SPECIFY) 1	39/
_____	
Private industry 1	40/
Other (SPECIFY) 1	41/
_____	

B. What are your main activities as an administrator--what do you do? (PROBE FOR CLARIFICATION ONLY)

C. What is your main title as an administrator?

9. Are you currently on the faculty of a medical school?

   Yes (ASK A-D). 1

   No 2

   A. At which medical school?

   B. What is your full title there?

   C. As a faculty member, are you on . . .

      full time salary, or 1

      part time salary, or 2

      are you not salaried? . . . 3

   D. As a faculty member, is your time spent . . .

      more with medical students, or 1

      more with house staff, or . 2

      with both groups about equally, or 3

      do you usually not work directly with either? . . . 4

10. Would you like to divide your profession time differently in order to spend more time in any of the activities we mention (that is, teaching, patient care, resear or administration)?

    Yes (ASK A) 1

    No 2

    A. In which ones would you like to spend more of your time?

       CODE AS MANY AS APPLY

       Teaching 1

       Patient care 1

       Research 1

       Administration 1

11. On the average, do you think you are working . . .

    too many hours, or 1

    just about the right number, or 2

    too few hours? 3

    DON'T KNOW 4

w for some questions on Medicare and other
sues.

What is your opinion about Medicare--
which pays for hospital and medical
care for those 65 or over--are you
personally . . .

strongly in favor, or 1   7/

somewhat in favor, or 2

somewhat opposed, or 3

strongly opposed? 4

DON'T KNOW 5

Do you recall--what was your opinion
about Medicare just before it was
passed by Congress in 1965. At that
time were you . . .

strongly in favor, or 1   8/

somewhat in favor, or 2

somewhat opposed, or 3

strongly opposed? 4

DON'T KNOW 5

Which one of these statements best
describes your overall opinion about
Medicare . . .

Medicare does not go far enough
in providing medical care for
older people, or 1   9/

it goes just far enough, or 2

it goes too far? 3

DON'T KNOW 4

All in all, how much has Medicare
actually affected your work . . .

a great deal, or (ASK A) 1   10/

a fair amount, or (ASK A) 2

very little, or 3

not at all? 4

DON'T KNOW 5

A. On the whole, has Medicare been . . .

a good thing for your work, or . . 1   11/

not such a good thing? 2

BOTH, NO DIFFERENCE . . 3

IF DOCTOR IN PATIENT CARE, ASK Q.16

16. About what percent of your patients
are 65 years or over? (Just your
best estimate)

Percent _____   12-14/

None 000

DON'T KNOW 999

ASK EVERYONE

17. In your opinion, as a result of Medicare,
are most doctors earning . . .

more money, or 1   15/

less money, or 2

hasn't Medicare made any
difference, or 3

do you have no idea?   . . 4

18. In your opinion, has the Federal government, under Medicare, affected the
individual doctor's professional
freedom . . .

a great deal, or 1   16/

a fair amount, or 2

very little, or 3

not at all, or 4

do you have no idea? 5

19. Of the doctors you know personally,
would you say . . .

most are in favor of
Medicare, ... 1   17/

-or-

most are opposed? 2

DON'T KNOW 3

-5-

20. Do you think the Federal government should be involved a great deal, a fair amount, very little, or not at all, in decisions about each of the following:

	A great deal	A fair amount	Very little	Not at all	DON'T KNOW	
A. The construction of hospitals	1	2	3	4	5	18
B. Medical school curricula	1	2	3	4	5	19
C. Priorities in biomedical research	1	2	3	4	5	20
D. Where doctors practice, by giving scholarships	1	2	3	4	5	21
E. Students' choice of specialty, by giving scholarships	1	2	3	4	5	22
F. Regulating the prescription drug industry	1	2	3	4	5	23
G. Providing medical care to poor people	1	2	3	4	5	24

21. Different proposals have been made in the past few years for a national health insurance plan covering everyone in the population. How well-informed do you feel you are about the various proposals? Are you . . .

very well informed, or 1   25/
fairly well informed, or 2
not well informed, or 3
not at all informed? 4

DON'T KNOW 5

22. On the whole, what is your opinion of some form of national health insurance? Are you . . .

strongly in favor, or 1   26/
somewhat in favor, or 2
somewhat opposed, or 3
strongly opposed? 4

DON'T KNOW 5

23. Do you think that some form of national health insurance is . . .

inevitable, (ASK A) 1   27
-or-
not inevitable? 2
DON'T KNOW . . . 3

A. About how many years do you think it will take . . .

less than a year 1   28
2 or 3 years 2
5 years 3
10 years, or 4
more than 10 years? 5

DON'T KNOW 6

f you were asked to advise a committee
lanning a national health insurance program . . .

4. Would you prefer a plan administered . . .

   by Blue Cross, Blue Shield, and
   private insurance companies, (ASK A) . .1   29/

               -or-

   by an agency of the Federal government like Health, Education, and
   Welfare? (ASK A) 2

               DON'T KNOW 3

   A. How strongly do you feel about
       this. . .

       strongly, or 1   30/

       not so strongly? 2

               DON'T KNOW 3

5. Assuming the Federal government covered
all poor people, would you prefer a
plan . . .

   financed by people who buy
   private health insurance with a
   tax-credit incentive, (ASK A) 1   31/

               -or-

   one financed by employer-employee
   contributions like Social
   Security? (ASK A) 2

               DON'T KNOW 3

   A. How strongly do you feel about
       this . . .

       strongly, or 1   32/

       not so strongly? 2

               DON'T KNOW 3

. Would you prefer a plan . . .

   under which the work of doctors is
   routinely reviewed by a panel of
   practicing doctors, (ASK A) 1   33/

               -or-

   a plan without such a system of
   reviews? (ASK A) 2

               DON'T KNOW 3

   A. How strongly do you feel about
       this . . .

       strongly, or 1   34/

       not so strongly? 2

               DON'T KNOW 3

27. Would you prefer a plan . . .

   that would support the development of
   prepaid group practice, where the patient
   gets complete care for a flat sum in
   advance (ASK A) 1   35/

               -or-

   one that would not support the
   development of prepaid group
   practice? (ASK A) 2

               DON'T KNOW 3

   A. How strongly do you feel about this . . .

       strongly, or 1   36/

       not so strongly? 2

               DON'T KNOW 3

28. Next--a question about how doctors should be
paid under national health insurance.
Would you be agreeable or not agreeable to . . .

	Agree-able	Not Agree-able	DON'T KNOW
A. a plan under which all doctors are paid an annual salary?	1	2	3 37/
B. a plan under which family doctors would be paid an annual amount for each patient they take care of?	1	2	3 38/
C. a plan under which all doctors would be paid a fixed fee for each service, negotiated by a committee on which physicians are represented?	1	2	3 39/
D. a plan under which all doctors would be paid their own customary fees for each service?	1	2	3 40/

-7-

IF DOCTOR IN PATIENT CARE, ASK Q.29

29. Under which of these methods do you
think you would earn the highest income . . .

an annual salary method, or 1   41/

an annual amount for each patient,or 2

fixed fees, or 3

your own customary fees? 4

DON'T KNOW . . . 5

IF DR. "NOT AT ALL INFORMED" ABOUT NAT'L
HEALTH INS. (Q.21) SKIP TO Q.31

30. Which one of the national health
insurance bills in Congress do
you prefer?

Kennedy bill, Kennedy-Griffith
bill, Health Security 1   42/

Nixon bill, Administration bill,
Byrnes-Bennett bill 2

AMA, Medicredit, Fulton-Broyhill
bill 3

Other (SPECIFY) 4

_____

Don't know enough about the bills · 5

Can't choose among bills 6

---

31. Assuming that a compromise of the various
national health insurance bills is
actually put into effect . . .

A. how much do you think it would
affect your work . . .

a great deal, or 1   43/

a fair amount, or 2

very little, or (SKIP TO C). . 3

not at all, or (SKIP TO C) . . 4

do you have no idea?
(SKIP TO C) 5

B. In general, would it be . . .

a good thing for your work,
or 1   44/

not such a good thing, or . . 2

do you have no idea? 3

C. Still assuming a compromise bill,
how do you think it would affect
the quality of care? Would most
people get . . .

better medical care, or 1   45/

not as good care, or 2

wouldn't it make any
difference, or 3

do you have no idea? 4

Q.31 CONTINUED IN THE NEXT COLUMN.

Q.31 CONTINUED

D. In the long run, would there be . . .

a great deal of unnecessary
hospitalization, or 1

a fair amount, or 2

very little, or 3

none at all, or 4

do you have no idea? 5

E. In the long run, would there be . . .

a great deal of unnecessary use
of doctors' services, or 1

a fair amount, or 2

very little, or 3

none at all, or 4

do you have no idea? 5

F. Under this same compromise program, do
you think most doctors would . . .

earn more money, or 1

less money, or 2

wouldn't it make any difference, or. 3

do you have no idea? 4

G. In your opinion, would the Federal government affect the individual doctor's
professional freedom . . .

a great deal, or 1

a fair amount, or 2

very little, or 3

not at all, or 4

do you have no idea? 5

---

32. Of the doctors you know personally, would
you say most are . . .

in favor of some form of national
health insurance, or 1

opposed to it? 2

DON'T KNOW 3

---

33. How much influence do you think the medical
profession will actually have on national
health insurance legislation . . .

a great deal, or 1

a fair amount, or 2

very little, or 3

none at all? 4

DON'T KNOW 5

-8-

I'm going to read some statements--and ask you if you agree strongly, agree only somewhat, disagree somewhat, or disagree strongly with each statement. The first one is . . .

	Agree Strongly	Agree Somewhat	Disagree Somewhat	Disagree Strongly	DON'T KNOW	
There are not enough physicians in this country.	1	2	3	4	5	52/
It is the responsibility of society, through its government, to provide everyone with the best available medical care, whether he can afford it or not.	1	2	3	4	5	53/
There are too many controls on the medical profession that interfere with taking care of patients.	1	2	3	4	5	54/
Regardless of shortcomings, the United States health care system is the best in the world.	1	2	3	4	5	55/
Large clinics are unable to give people individualized care.	1	2	3	4	5	56/
A doctor's conscience is more important for the quality of medicine he practices, than are reviews of his work by other doctors.	1	2	3	4	5	57/
Decisions about the organization of health care should be entirely in the hands of the medical profession.	1	2	3	4	5	58/
It is the responsibility of society, through its government, to guarantee full employment.	1	2	3	4	5	59/
The government should play a bigger part in the economic life of the nation in order to distribute income more equally.	1	2	3	4	5	60/
Poverty could almost be done away with if we made certain basic changes in our social and economic system.	1	2	3	4	5	61/
The United States needs a complete restructuring of its basic institutions.	1	2	3	4	5	62 /

-9-

BEGIN DECK 44

35. A. Considering the following list of
arrangements for practicing medicine,
which one, in your opinion, is likely
to lead to the <u>best medical care</u>?
READ ENTIRE LIST. CODE IN COLUMN "A"
BELOW.

	A. Best Medical Care	B. Most Desir- able	C. Least Desir- able
Solo practice	1 8/	1 9/	1 10/
Partnership of two physicians	2	2	2
A <u>small</u> group of 3 to 5 physicians, in <u>one</u> specialty	3	3	3
A <u>small</u>, multi-specialty group	4	4	4
A <u>large</u> group of 20 physicians or more <u>not</u> in a hospital, or	5	5	5
A <u>large</u> group based in a hospital?	6	6	6
DON'T KNOW	7	7	7

B. Considering the same list of arrange-
ments--suppose your income in all of
these were the same --which one would
you consider <u>most desirable</u> for yourself? CODE IN COLUMN "B" ABOVE.

C. And which one would be <u>least desirable</u>
for yourself? CODE IN COLUMN "C" ABOVE.

36. Assuming that the physician gets paid a fee
for each service, which of the following
systems do you prefer . . .

one of <u>simple prepayment</u>, that
is, which provides complete care
to a family for a flat sum in
advance, or 1   11/

one of <u>modified prepayment</u> where
the patient must pay a <u>small fee</u>--
say a dollar or two--for each
service, or 2

one in which the patient pays
for each service and is <u>completely
reimbursed</u> by a third party, or . . . 3

one in which the patient pays the
whole fee for each service <u>without
being reimbursed</u>? 4

DON'T KNOW 5

A. How strongly do you feel about this . . .

strongly, or 1   12/

not so strongly? 2

DON'T KNOW 3

37. The use of nurse-practitioners and physicians'
assistants has been proposed as one way to
make better use of doctors' time.

For each of the following duties, please
tell me whether you think it is appropriate
or not for such persons, assuming that they
are properly trained and working under the
supervision of a physician.

	Yes, Appropriate	No, not Appropriate	DON KNO
A. Taking preliminary histories.	1	2	3
B. Performing routine physical examina-tions.	1	2	3
C. Differentiating between functional and organic murmurs.	1	2	3
D. Deciding if suturing is necessary.	1	2	3
E. Treating super-ficial corneal abrasions.	1	2	3
F. Deciding whether a patient with what appears to be a minor complaint should be seen by a doctor.	1	2	3
G. Deciding what allergy tests to do.	1	2	3
H. Doing allergy tests.	1	2	3
I. Diagnosing throat conditions.	1	2	3
J. Deciding whether to prescribe an anti-biotic for a sore throat.	1	2	3
K. Prescribing medication for minor pain relief.	1	2	3
L. Reading simple chest X-rays in a screening program.	1	2	3
M. Doing minor suturing.	1	2	3
N. Counselling a diabetic patient about his diet.	1	2	3
O. Doing routine physical examinations on cardiac patients in follow-ups.	1	2	3
P. Doing routine well-baby follow-ups.	1	2	3
Q. Doing routine pre-natal check-ups on the mother.	1	2	3
R. Performing uncom-plicated deliveries <u>in the hospital</u>.	1	2	3

-10-

38. Would you use such a person in your practice, or not (if you were in practice)?

Yes 1   31/

No 2

DON'T KNOW 3

39. More and more reviews are being made of doctors' work in hospitals by other doctors. What is your opinion of such a trend--are you . . .

strongly in favor, or 1   32/

somewhat in favor, or 2

somewhat opposed, or 3

strongly opposed   4

DON'T KNOW 5

40. Now, how about reviews of doctors' work in their offices by other doctors--in general, are you . . .

strongly in favor, or(ASK A-C). 1   33/

somewhat in favor, or(ASK A-C). 2

somewhat opposed, or 3

strongly opposed? 4

DON'T KNOW 5

IF "IN FAVOR", ASK A, B, AND C

A. How would you feel about a committee that includes physicians not in patient care, to review doctors' work in their offices. Would you be . . .

agreeable, or 1   34/

not agreeable? 2

DON'T KNOW 3

B. How about a committee of physicans representing the State health department. Would you be . . .

agreeable, or 1   35/

not agreeable? 2

DON'T KNOW 3

C. How about a committee that includes some non-physicians, representing consumers. Would you be . . .

agreeable, or. 1   36/

not agreeable? 2

DON'T KNOW 3

41. For each of the following statements, please tell me if you agree strongly, agree only somewhat, disagree somewhat, or disagree strongly.

A. The practice of medicine is both an "art" and a "science" but it should be more like a science than like an art.

Agree strongly 1   37/

Agree somewhat 2

Disagree somewhat 3

Disagree strongly 4

DON'T KNOW 5

B. In general, the doctor who bases his diagnosis mainly on clinical signs is likely to give better medical care than one who bases his diagnosis mainly on laboratory tests.

Agree strongly 1   38/

Agree somewhat 2

Disagree somewhat 3

Disagree strongly 4

DON'T KNOW 5

C. In general, a doctor's skill in the technical details of diagnosis and treatment is more important for the quality of medicine he practices than his skill in establishing a personal relationship with his patients.

Agree strongly 1   39/

Agree somewhat 2

Disagree somewhat 3

Disagree strongly 4

DON'T KNOW 5

D. Medical schools should put more emphasis on preventive medicine in their curricula.

Agree strongly 1   40/

Agree somewhat 2

Disagree somewhat 3

Disagree strongly 4

DON'T KNOW 5

E. The medical value of annual health examinations for people who are not sick has been exaggerated.

Agree strongly 1   41/

Agree somewhat 2

Disagree somewhat 3

Disagree strongly 4

DON'T KNOW 5

CONTINUED ON NEXT PAGE

-11-

Q.41 CONTINUED

F. It is a good idea for medical students and nursing students to take some courses together.

　Agree strongly . . . . 1　42/

　Agree somewhat 2

　Disagree somewhat 3

　Disagree strongly 4

　　　　DON'T KNOW 5

G. Doctors generally do not have enough respect for nurses.

　Agree strongly . . . . 1　43/

　Agree somewhat 2

　Disagree somewhat 3

　Disagree strongly 4

　　　　DON'T KNOW 5

H. Physicians should rely more on their personal clinical experience in treating their patients than on the results of controlled clinical studies by others.

　Agree strongly . . . . 1　44/

　Agree somewhat 2

　Disagree somewhat 3

　Disagree strongly 4

　　　　DON'T KNOW 5

I. On the whole, it is more important for the doctor to choose the treatment that helps the patient rather than to know why the treatment works.

　Agree strongly . . . . 1　45/

　Agree somewhat 2

　Disagree somewhat 3

　Disagree strongly 4

　　　　DON'T KNOW 5

J. It is generally better for the practitioner to prescribe something for each patient-- such as medication or some other treatment-- rather than to prescribe nothing at all.

　Agree strongly . . . . 1　46/

　Agree somewhat 2

　Disagree somewhat 3

　Disagree strongly 4

　　　　DON'T KNOW 5

Q.41 CONTINUED

K. Good medicine requires more than just treating people who come for care; it requires that doctors work in programs to improve social conditions.

　Agree strongly . . . . 1　47

　Agree somewhat 2

　Disagree somewhat 3

　Disagree strongly 4

　　　　DON'T KNOW 5

L. The practitioner's main responsibility is to his patients rather than to the community as a whole.

　Agree strongly . . . . 1　48

　Agree somewhat 2

　Disagree somewhat 3

　Disagree strongly 4

　　　　DON'T KNOW 5

M. One should not become a doctor unless he or she is willing to work long and irregular hours.

　Agree strongly . . . . 1　49

　Agree somewhat 2

　Disagree somewhat 3

　Disagree strongly 4

　　　　DON'T KNOW 5

42. As a practicing physician, (are you/would you be) . . .

　more inclined to try out new forms of treatment, or . . . . . . .1　50

　more inclined to rely on accepted forms of treatment? 2

　　　　DON'T KNOW 3

43. How much uncertainty do you think there is in doctors' decisions about treatment . . .

　a great deal, or . . . . .1　51

　a fair amount, or 2

　very little? 3

　　　　DON'T KNOW 4

44. All other things being equal, would you prefer . . .

　treating a patient whose condi- tion requires your consulting with other doctors, or . . . . . . .1　52

　one whose condition does not? . . .2

　　　　DON'T KNOW 3

-12-

. "Community participation" in health care can
mean different things.

A. In setting goals and priorities for the
hospital, do you think local residents,
elected to hospital boards by the
community, should have . . .

        voting power, or 1   53/

        an advisory role only, or . . . 2

        should not be involved
        at all? 3

                DON'T KNOW 4

B. How about in the selection of professional
staff -- do you think these elected
residents should have . . .

        voting power, or 1   54/

        an advisory role only, or . . . 2

        should not be involved
        at all? 3

                DON'T KNOW 4

. In your opinion, is it ever justifiable
for physicians to go on strike, or not?

        Justifiable 1   55/

        Not justifiable 2

                DON'T KNOW 3

. The allocation of scarce resources poses
difficult problems for the medical
profession. Suppose you had to decide
how to spend one and a half million
dollars a year in a health budget.
Would you be more likely to spend the
money . . .

    for hemodyalysis for 100
    adolescent patients who would
    otherwise die,. 1   56/

            -or-

    for medical care for 10,000 people
    who would otherwise get no care? . . . 2

                DON'T KNOW 3

. A. Do you feel that . . .

    a terminally ill patient who
    gives no indication of wanting
    to know should be told about
    his prognosis,. 1   57/

            -or-

    do you feel that he should not
    be told? 2

                DON'T KNOW 3

Q. 48 CONTINUED IN NEXT COLUMN

48. B. In your opinion, should a patient with
a terminal illness . . .

        be permitted to refuse further
        treatment that will prolong
        his life 1   58/

                -or-

        should he not be permitted to
        refuse further treatment?. 2

                DON'T KNOW 3

C. In general, how likely (are you/would
you be) to recommend to the family of
a comatose terminally ill patient that
treatment be continued to prolong his
life . . .

        very likely, or 1   59/

        somewhat likely, or 2

        not likely? 3

                DON'T KNOW 4

D. About how many terminally ill patients
have you taken care of during the past
year?   # _____ 60-61/

        NONE 00

        98 or more 98

                DON'T KNOW . . . 99
                                        62/R

49. Conducting research on human beings also
raises ethical problems.

In general, would you be . . .

        more likely to support research
        with a risk to the patient, but
        with a chance that its results
        will benefit other patients,. . . .1   63/

                -or-

        more likely to oppose such
        research? 2

                DON'T KNOW 3

50. Recent abortion reform laws allow a woman
to have an abortion if she and her doctor
agree. Are you . . .

        strongly in favor of such
        laws, or 1   64/

        somewhat in favor, or. 2

        somewhat opposed, or 3

        strongly opposed? 4

                DON'T KNOW 5

-13-

BEGIN DECK 45

51. About how old were you when you definitely decided to go into medicine?

15 or under . . . 1   20 or 21 4   20/

16 or 17 2   22 or over . . . 5

18 or 19 3   DON'T KNOW . 6

52. A. While you were in medical school, did you ever have any doubts that medicine was the right profession for you--would you say you had . . .

serious doubts, or 1   21/

slight doubts, or 2

no doubts at all? 3

DON'T KNOW 4

B. How about at the present time--do you have any doubts that medicine is the right profession for you-- would you say you have . . .

serious doubts, or 1   22/

slight doubts, or 2

no doubts at all? 3

DON'T KNOW 4

53. A. Which of the following gives you the most satisfaction . . . CODE IN COLUMN "A" BELOW.

	A. Most Satisfaction	B. Next Most Satisfaction
Work,	1 23/	1 24/
Family life,	2	2
Recreational and cultural activities,	3	3
Religious activities, or	4	4
Civic activities.	5	5
DON'T KNOW	6	6

B. Which gives you the next most satisfaction? CODE IN COLUMN "B" ABOVE.

54. A. In your decision to go into medicine, how important was each of the following . . . very important, somewhat important, or not at all important?

CIRCLE ONE CODE FOR EACH ITEM IN COLUMN "A" BELOW

	Very Important	Somewhat Important	A. Not at all Important	DON'T KNOW	IN DECISION B. Most Important	IN DECISION C. 2nd most Imp.	NOW D. Most Imp.	NOW E. 2nd Most Imp.
1) Making a lot of money?	1	2	3	4 25/	1 32/	1 33/	1 34/	1 35/
2) Opportunities to be original and creative?	1	2	3	4 26/	2	2	2	2
3) Opportunities to be helpful to others or useful to society?	1	2	3	4 27/	3	3	3	3
4) Working in a demanding field that brings out your best efforts?	1	2	3	4 28/	4	4	4	4
5) Freedom from supervision in your work?	1	2	3	4 29/	5	5	5	5
6) Opportunity to work with people rather than things?	1	2	3	4 30/	6	6	6	6
7) Having prestige in the community?	1	2	3	4 31/	7	7	7	7
					D.K.8	D.K.8	D.K.8	D.K.8

B. Which one of these was most important in your decision to go into medicine? CIRCLE THE ITEM NUMBER IN COLUMN "B" ABOVE.

C. Which one of these was second most important? CIRCLE THE ITEM NUMBER IN COLUMN "C" ABOVE.

D. How about the present -- which one of these is most important now? CIRCLE THE ITEM NUMBER IN COLUMN "D" ABOVE.

E. Which one is second most important now? CIRCLE THE ITEM NUMBER IN COLUMN "E" ABOVE.

-14-

ould you say that medicine is . . .

the only career that could really
satisfy you, or 1   36/

that it is one of several that you
could find almost equally
satisfying, or 2

can you think of other careers
that would be more satisfying
to you? 3

DON'T KNOW   . . . 4

---

o you think medical schools are spending . . .

too much time on the basic
sciences, or 1   37/

just about the right amount, or . .2

not enough time? 3

DON'T KNOW 4

---

s a practicing physician, (do/would)
ou get more personal satisfaction from . . .

solving a relatively simple
medical problem for a patient
who expresses great
appreciation, ... 1   38/

-or-

solving a very complicated
problem for a patient who
expresses no appreciation
whatever? 2

DON'T KNOW . . . 3

. The emphasis on pathology in medical
training makes it difficult for
doctors to think of each patient
as an individual. How about you--
most of the time do you think of
a patient . . .

as an individual, or 1   39/

as a disease entity? 2

DON'T KNOW 3

. Compared with when you started
medical school, are you . . .

more likely now to think of
each patient as a disease
entity, or 1   40/

less likely, or 2

has there been no change? . . . 3

DON'T KNOW . . . 4

---

59. In general, how much does the possibility of
a malpractice suit affect how doctors practice
medicine--would you say . . .

a great deal, or 1   41/

a fair amount, or 2

very little, or 3

not at all? 4

DON'T KNOW 5

IF RESPONDENT IS IN PATIENT CARE, ASK Q's. 60 & 61

60. How about you, yourself--does the
possibility of a malpractice suit
affect how you practice medicine--
would you say . . .

a great deal, or 1   42/

a fair amount, or 2

very little, or 3

not at all? 4

DON'T KNOW 5

---

61. How satisfied are you with the amount of time
you can spend with each patient . . .

very satisfied, or 1   43/

somewhat satisfied, or 2

not satisfied? 3

DON'T KNOW 4

ASK EVERYONE

62. Computers are used in a variety of ways
in the practice of medicine.

Would you say computers right now are very
useful, or somewhat useful, or not useful --
or do you have no idea . . .

	Very Useful	Somewhat Useful	Not Useful	No Idea	
A. in keeping patients' medical records?	1	2	3	4	44/
B. in the diagnosis of symptoms?	1	2	3	4	45/
C. in multiphasic screening programs for the early detection of disease?	1	2	3	4	46/
D. in monitoring patients in intensive care units?	1	2	3	4	47/

48-49/R

63. Do you belong to the . . .

FOR EACH "YES" IN QUESTION 63, ASK QUESTIONS 64 AND 65

		63.			64. Have you attended any meetings of that organization in the past 12 months?			65. In the past 5 years have you been an officer or committee chairman in that organization?		
		Yes	No		Yes		No	Yes		No
A.	county medical society?	1	2	50/	1		2 56/	1		2 6:
B.	state medical society?	1	2	51/	1		2 57/	1		2 6.
C.	American Medical Association?	1	2	52/	1		2 58/	1		2 6
D.	Any other professional societies? IF YES, SPECIFY THE NAMES, ONE IN EACH SPACE.	1	2	53/	1		2 59/	1		2 6.
E.		1	2	54/	1		2 60/	1		2 6
F.		1	2	55/	1		2 61/	1		2 6

79-80/4

BEGIN DECK 46

66. Have you ever had an article published in a professional journal?

Yes (ASK A) 1   8/

No 2

A. How many?   _____ 9-10/

98 or more 98

DON'T KNOW .99

67. Thinking about issues in the organization of health care, does the American Medical Association represent your personal opinion . . .

on most matters, or 1   11/

on some, or 2

on hardly any? 3

DON'T KNOW . .4

68. Should doctors who disagree with the policies of the A.M.A. . . .

try to change the organization by working within it, or 1   12/

by working with another organization? 2

DON'T KNOW . 3

69. Comparing yourself to most physicians you know, do you take . . .

more active interest in issues in the organization of health care, or 1   1

less active interest, or 2

about the same? 3

DON'T KNOW 4

70. In recent years some medical students and doctors have used "activist" methods to express views on issues ranging from higher stipends to protest against the war. Regardless of the issue, do you feel it is proper or not proper for physicians . . .

	Yes, Proper	No, not Proper	DON'T KNOW
A. to place pamphlets and posters in their waiting rooms?	1	2	3 1
B. to wear buttons with slogans while on duty?	1	2	3 1
C. to participate as doctors in marches and other demonstrations?	1	2	3
D. to disrupt medical society or other meetings?	1	2	3

A. With whom do you spend more of your
free time . . .

    with doctors, or. 1   18/

    with people in other
work?. 2

B. Among your three closest friends, is
any of them a doctor?

    Yes (ASK (1)). 1   19/

    No 2

  (1) How many? _____   20/

. Which is more important to you . . .

    having the respect of the
people in your community, or 1   21/

    having the respect of
other physicians? 2

          DON'T KNOW. .3

. a few background questions.

. What is your age? YEARS:_____   22-23/

. Are you . . .

    married, or (ASK A) . . . 1   24/

    separated, or 2

    divorced, or 3

    widowed, or 4

    single, never married? . 5

A. Is this your first marriage?

    Yes 1   25/

    No 2

EVER-MARRIED, ASK QUESTIONS 75 AND 76.

. How many children do you have?

         _____   26/

    None 0

ANY CHILDREN: A. How old is the oldest?

      YEARS:_____   27-28/

. (Is/Was) your spouse a physician?

    Yes 1   29/

    No 2

. What is your race?

    White 1   30/

    Black 2

    Oriental 3

    Other (SPECIFY) 4

78. In what country were you born?

    United States 1   31/

    Canada 2

    Other (SPECIFY) 3

79. Was either of your parents born outside the
United States? (Which one?)

    Yes, mother 1   32/

    Yes, father 2

    Yes, both 3

    No, neither 4

80. What state did you live in most of the time
before you started medical school?

    Did not live in the United States. 00 **33-34/**

Alabama	01	Missouri	26
Alaska	02	Montana	27
Arizona	03	Nebraska	28
Arkansas	04	Nevada	29
California	05	New Hampshire.	30
Colorado	06	New Jersey	31
Connecticut	07	New Mexico	32
Delaware	08	New York	33
D. of Col.	09	North Carolina	34
Florida	10	North Dakota	35
Georgia	11	Ohio	36
Hawaii	12	Oklahoma	37
Idaho	13	Oregon	38
Illinois	14	Pennsylvania	39
Indiana	15	Rhode Island	40
Iowa	16	South Carolina	41
Kansas	17	South Dakota	42
Kentucky	18	Tennessee	43
Louisiana	19	Texas	44
Maine	20	Utah	45
Maryland	21	Vermont	46
Massachusetts	22	Virginia	47
Michigan	23	Washington	48
Minnesota	24	West Virginia	49
Mississippi	25	Wisconsin	50
		Wyoming	51

81. In what religion were you brought up?

    Protestant 1   35/

    Roman Catholic 2

    Jewish 3

    Other (SPECIFY) 4

    None 5

238   Physicians and Social Change

82. What is your __present__ religious affiliation?

Protestant 1   36/
Roman Catholic 2
Jewish 3
Other (SPECIFY) · · · · · 4

_____

None 5

83. Do you consider yourself . . .

deeply religious, or 1   37/
moderately religious, or 2
largely indifferent to
religion, or 3
basically opposed to
religion? 4

DON'T KNOW 5

84. What was the last grade or year in
school your father completed?

Eighth grade or less 1   38/
Some high school 2
High school graduate 3
Business or technical school
after high school 4
Some college 5
College graduate 6
More than college 7
Other (SPECIFY)

_____ 8

DON'T KNOW 9

85. A. What kind of work did your father do
__most__ of the time when you were in
your teens? What exactly did he do?

Father deceased at that
time (SKIP TO Q.88) 1   39/
Father a physician
(GO TO Q.86) 2

B. What industry was that in?

40-42/

C. Was he . . .

self-employed, or 1   43/
did he work for someone
else? 2

44/R

86. Did your father consider himself a . . .

Democrat 1   45/
-or-
Republican 2
-or-
some other party? (SPECIFY) . . . 3

_____

DON'T KNOW 4
Father never lived in the
United States or not a citizen
of the United States 5

87. In his political thinking would you describe
your father as . . .

radical left, or 1   46/
liberal, or 2
middle-of-the-road, or 3
conservative, or 4
radical right? 5

DON'T KNOW . . . 6

88. Do you consider yourself . . .

a strong Democrat, or 1   47/
a not very strong Democrat, or . . .2
a strong Republican, or 3
a not very strong Republican, or . .4
an independent? (ASK A) 5
Other (SPECIFY)_____ 6
Not a citizen of the United
States (SKIP TO Q.90) 7

DON'T KNOW 8

IF INDEPENDENT: A. Do you identify more
closely with the . . .

Democratic party 1   48/
-or-
Republican party? 2

DON'T KNOW 3

-18-

When you started medical school, <u>did</u> you consider yourself . . .

 a strong Democrat, or 1   49/

 a not very strong Democrat, or . 2

 a strong Republican, or 3

 a not very strong Republican, or 4

 an independent? (ASK A) 5

 Other (SPECIFY) 6

 Not a citizen of the U.S. 7

     DON'T KNOW . . . 8

IF INDEPENDENT: A. Did you identify more closely with the . . .

 Democratic party 1 50/
     -or-
 Republican party? 2

    DON'T KNOW 3

In your political thinking, do you consider yourself as . . .

 radical left, or 1 51/

 liberal, or 2

 middle-of-the-road, or 3

 conservative, or 4

 radical right? 5

    DON'T KNOW . . . 6

Compared to when you started medical school, do you consider yourself politically . . .

 more conservative now, or 1 52/

 less conservative, or 2

 has there been no change? 3

    DON'T KNOW 4

Which one of the following comes closest to describing the social class your parents belonged to when you were in your teens . . .

 upper class, or 1 53/

 upper middle class, or 2

 lower middle class, or 3

 working class, or 4

 lower class? 5

    DON'T KNOW 6

93. What is your realistic estimate of your final standing in medical school? Were you in the . . .

 top quarter, or 1 54/

 2nd quarter, or 2

 3rd quarter, or 3

 4th quarter, or 4

 do you have no idea? 5

94. Were you in debt when you graduated from medical school--including debts to your family that you felt obliged to pay back?

 Yes 1 55/

 No 2

95. A. In which of these following groups was your net professional income in 1972, that is, after expenses, but before taxes. Just these broad groups . . .

 Under $20,000 . . . . .1 56/

 $20,000 to $29,999 2

 $30,000 to $39,999 3

 $40,000 to $49,999 4

 $50,000 to $59,999 5

 $60,000 to $79,999 6

 $80,000 or more? 7

 B. About what percent of this was salary?

 None 1 57/

 1-24% 2

 25-49% 3

 50-74% 4

 75-99% 5

 100% 6

    DON'T KNOW . . . 7

96. How satisfied are you with your professional income -- are you . . .

 very satisfied, or 1 58/

 somewhat satisfied, or 2

 not satisfied? 3

    DON'T KNOW . . .4

-19-

97. In general, how happy are you with your
     present career within medicine -- are
     you . . .

                very happy, or 1   59/

                somewhat happy, or . . . 2

                not happy? 3

                       DON'T KNOW . . 4

                                   79-80/46

Thank you very much.

Would you like to make any comments about
any of the things we've talked about?

BEGIN DECK 4?

INTERVIEWER REMARKS

A. Time interview ended: _____

B. How long did this interview take?

                    _____ minutes 8-1(

C. How many sessions?   _____   1)

D. Month and date, interview completed?

    Month: Feb. . . . 2 12/ Date _____ 13-?
            Mar. . . . 3
            Apr. . . . 4
            May. . . . 5
            June . . . 6
            July . . . 7

E. Was the doctor . . .

            very cooperative 1   1.
            fairly cooperative 2
            fairly hostile 3
            very hostile? 4

F. Did the doctor request a copy of the results?

            Yes 1   1.
            No 2

G. Interviewer's I.D. __ __ __ __ __   17-2

    Interviewer's Signature:

    _____

H. Any other general comments about this
    interview? (IF NOT ENOUGH ROOM, CONTINUE
    ON BACK PAGE)

References

Abelson, R. P., Aronson, E., McGuire, W. J., Newcomb, T. M., Rosenberg, M. J., and Tannenbaum, P. H. *Theories of Cognitive Consistency: A Sourcebook.* Chicago: Rand McNally, 1968.

Abramson, P. R. *Generational Change in American Politics.* Lexington, MA: Lexington Books, 1975.

Abramson, P. R. *Political Attitudes in America.* San Francisco: Freeman, 1983.

Adams, B. N., and Meidam, M. T. Economics, family structure, and college attendance. *Am. J. Sociol.* 74:230–239, 1968.

Adams, S. Trends in occupational origins of physicians. *Am. Sociol. Rev.* 18:404–409, 1953.

Adelson, J. *Handbook of Adolescent Psychology.* New York: Wiley, 1980.

Alford, R. *Party and Society: The Anglo-American Democracies.* Chicago: Rand McNally, 1963.

Alford, R. *Health Care Politics: Ideological and Interest Group Barriers to Reform.* Chicago: University of Chicago Press, 1975.

Allport, G. W. *The Nature of Prejudice.* Cambridge, MA: Addison-Wesley, 1954.

Altman, S. H., and Blendon, R. (Eds.). *Medical Technology: The Culprit Behind Health Care Costs? Proceedings of the 1977 Sun Valley Forum on National Health.* DHEW Publication No. (PHS) 79-3216. Washington, DC: U.S. Government Printing Office, 1979.

American Medical Association. The Voluntary Way Is the American Way, undated.

American Medical Association. Opinions and Reports of the Judicial Council. Chicago, 1969.

American Medical Association. Does the AMA Really Represent Your Interests? Undated [ca 1975].

American Medical Association. *1973 American Medical Directory.* Chicago, 1974.

American Medical Association. Public Attitudes toward Health Care and Health Care Issues. Chicago, 1979.

American Medical Association, Physicians' Perceptions of Issues in Health Care and Medicine. Chicago, 1981a.

American Medical Association. Public Attitudes toward Health Care and Health Care Issues. Chicago, 1981b.

American Medical Association. Medical Groups in the U.S., 1980. Chicago, 1982a.

American Medical Association. AMA Cost-Effectiveness Plan: 1982 and Beyond, Chicago, 1982b.

American Medical Association. Physician Characteristics and Distribution in the U.S., 1982 edition. Chicago, 1983a.

American Medical Association. Physician Opinion on Health Care Issues, 1983b.

American Medical Association. AMA Cost-Effectiveness Plan: 1984 and Beyond, 1984.

The AMA House of Delegates: Does it really speak for American medicine? *Medical World News* 12:37–48, June 18, 1971.

The American Medical Association: Power, purpose, and politics in organized medicine. *Yale Law J.* 63:938–1022, 1954.

Back, K. W., Phillips, B. S., Coker, R. E., Jr., and Donnelly, T. G. Public health as a career in medicine: Secondary choice within a profession. *Am. Sociol. Rev.* 23:533–541, 1958.

Badgley, R. F., and Wolfe, S. *Doctors' Strike: Medical Care and Conflict in Saskatchewan.* New York: Atherton Press, 1967.

Ball, H. V., Simpson, G. E., and Ikeda, K. Law and social change: Sumner reconsidered. *Am. J. Sociol.* 67:532–540, 1962.

Barhydt-Wezenaar, N. Nursing. In Jonas, S. (Ed.), *Health Care Delivery in the United States.* Second Edition. New York: Springer, 1981, pp. 96–125.

Barr, J. K., and Steinberg, M. K. Organizational structure and professional norms in an alternative health care setting: Physicians in health maintenance organizations. *J. Sociol. & Social Welfare* 7:341–358, 1980.

Becker, H. S. Personal change in adult life. *Sociometry* 27:40–53, 1964.

Becker, H. S., and Geer, B. Latent culture: A note on the theory of latent social roles. *Administrative Science Q.* 5:304–313, 1960.

Becker, H. S., Geer, B., Hughes, E. C., and Strauss, A. L. *Boys in White.* Chicago: University of Chicago Press, 1961.

Ben-David, J. The professional role of the physician in bureaucratized medicine: A study in role conflict. *Hum. Relations* 11:255–274, 1958.

Ben-David, J. Professions in the class systems of present-day societies. *Current Sociol.* 12:247–255, 1963–64.

Bendix, R. *Higher Civil Servants in American Society: A Study of the Social Origins, the Careers, and the Power-Position of Higher Federal Administration.* Boulder, CO: University of Colorado Press, Series in Sociology No. 1, 1949.

Bendix, R., and Lipset, S. M. (Eds.). *Class, Status, and Power.* New York: Free Press, 1966.

Bengtson, V. L., and Cutler, N. E. Generations and intergenerational relations: Perspectives on age groups and social change. In Binstock, R. H. and Shanas, E. (Eds.), *Handbook of Aging and the Social Sciences.* New York: Van Nostrand Reinhold, 1976, pp. 130–159.

Benham, L., and Benham, A. The impact of incremental medical services on health status. In Andersen, R., Kravitz, J., and Anderson, O. W. (Eds.), *Equity in Health Services: Empirical Analyses in Social Policy.* Cambridge, MA: Ballinger, 1975.

Berelson, B., and Steiner, G. A. *Human Behavior: An Inventory of Scientific Findings.* New York: Harcourt, Brace & World, 1964.

Berelson, B. P., Lazarsfeld, P. F., and McPhee, W. N. *Voting.* Chicago: University of Chicago Press, 1954.

Berger, M. *Equality by Statute.* New York: Columbia University Press, 1954.

Berki, S. E. Health care policy: Lessons from the past and issues of the future. *Ann. Am. Acad. of Political and Social Sciences* 468:231–246, 1983.

Berkowitz, L., and Walker, N. Laws and moral judgments. *Sociometry* 30:410–422, 1967.

Berman, D. E., and Gertman, P. M. Cost containment and quality assurance: The potential and performance of the Professional Standards Review Organization Program. In Altman, S. H. and Sapolsky, H. M. (Eds.), *Federal Health Programs: Problems and Prospects.* Lexington, MA: Lexington Books, 1981, pp. 43–61.

Blalock, H. M. *Social Statistics*, revised second edition. New York: McGraw-Hill, 1979.

Blau, P., and Scott, R. W. *Formal Organizations*. San Francisco: Chandler, 1961.

Bloom, S. W. The sociology of medical education: Some comments on the state of a field. *Milbank Memorial Fund Q.* 43:143-184, 1965.

Bloom, S. W. Socialization for the physician's role: A review of some contributions of research to theory. In Shapiro, E. C. and Loewenstein, L. M. (Eds.), *Becoming a Physician*. Cambridge, MA: Ballinger, 1979, pp. 3-52.

Bonfield, A. E. The role of legislation in eliminating racial discrimination. *Race* 7:107-122, 1965.

Bosk, C. L. *Forgive and Remember: Managing Medical Failure*. Chicago: University of Chicago Press, 1979.

Bottomore, T. B., and Rubel, M. (Eds.). *Karl Marx: Selected Writings in Sociology and Social Philosophy*. London: Watts & Co., 1956.

Braungart, R. G. Youth movements. In Adelson, J. (Ed.), *Handbook of Adolescent Psychology*. New York: Wiley, 1980, pp. 560-597.

Breed, W., and Ktsanes, T. Pluralistic ignorance in the process of opinion formation. *Publ. Opinion Q.* 25:382-392, 1961.

Brimm, O. G., Jr., and Wheeler, S. *Socialization After Childhood: Two Essays*. New York: Wiley, 1966.

Brint, S. The political attitudes of professionals. In Turner, R. H. and Short, J. F., Jr. (Eds.), *Annual Review of Sociology*. Palo Alto: Annual Reviews, 1985, pp. 389-414.

Brown, L. Health policy in the Reagan administration: A critical appraisal. *Bull. N Y Acad. Med.* 59:33-40, 1983.

Bruhn, J. G., and Parsons, A. O. Medical student attitudes toward four medical specialties. *J. Med. Educ.* 39:40-49, 1964.

Brunswick, A. F. What generation gap? *Social Problems* 17:358-371, 1970.

Bucher, R., and Strauss, A. Professions in process. *Am. J. Sociol.* 66:325-334, 1961.

Bucher, R., and Stelling, J. G. *Becoming Professional*. Beverly Hills, CA: Sage Publications, 1977.

Burrow, J. G. *AMA: Voice of American Medicine*. Baltimore, MD: Johns Hopkins Press, 1963.

Bush, D. M., and Simmons, R. G. Socialization processes over the life course. In Rosenberg, M. and Turner, R. L. (Eds.), *Social Psychology: Sociological Perspectives*. New York: Basic Books, 1981, pp. 133-164.

Bynder, H. Physicians choose psychiatrists: Medical social structure and patterns of choice. *J. Health and Hum. Behavior* 6:83-91, 1965.

Cafferata, G. L. Medical specialties and American national health policy: 1967-1973. Ph.D. Dissertation, University of Chicago, 1974.

California Medical Association. Triennial survey of medical students and recent graduates: 1981. San Francisco, Oct. 1982.

Campbell, A., Converse, P. E., Miller, W. E., and Stokes, D. E. *The American Voter*. New York: Wiley, 1960.

Campbell, D. T. From description to experimentation: Interpreting trends as quasi-experiments. In Harris, C. W. (Ed.), *Problems in Measuring Change*. Madison, WI: University of Wisconsin Press, 1963, pp. 212-242.

Campbell, D. T., and Clayton, K. N. Avoiding regression effects in panel studies of communication impact. *Studies in Public Communication* 3:99-118, 1961.

Campbell, E. Q. The attitude effects of educational desegregation in a southern community: A methodological study in scale analysis. Ph.D. Dissertation, Vanderbilt University, 1956.

Campbell, E. Q. Some social psychological correlates of direction in attitude change. *Social Forces* 36:335–340, 1958.

Campion, F. *The AMA and U.S. Health Policy Since 1940.* Chicago: Chicago Review Press, 1984.

Cantril, H. *Gauging Public Opinion.* Princeton: Princeton University Press, 1947.

Carlin, J. E. *Lawyers' Ethics: A Survey of the New York City Bar.* New York: Russell Sage Foundation, 1966.

Chase, H. C. Infant mortality and its concomitants, 1960–1972. *Medical Care* 15(8):662–674, 1977.

Clark, K. B. Desegregation: An appraisal of the evidence. *J. Social Issues* 9:1–76, 1953.

Coe, R., Pepper, M., and Mattis, M. The "new" medical student: Another view. *J. Med. Educ.* 52:89–98, 1977.

Cohn, W. The politics of American Jews. In M. Sklare (Ed.), *The Jews: Social Patterns of an American Group.* Glencoe, IL: Free Press, 1958, pp. 614–626.

Cole, J. *Fair Science: Women in the Scientific Community.* New York: Free Press, 1979.

Cole, J., and Cole, S. *Social Stratification in Science.* Chicago: University of Chicago Press, 1973.

Cole, J., and Zuckerman, H. The emergence of a scientific specialty: The self-exemplifying case of the sociology of science. In Coser, L. A. (Ed.), *The Idea of Social Structure: Papers in Honor of Robert K. Merton.* New York: Harcourt Brace Jovanovich, 1975, pp. 139–174.

Colombotos, J. Sources of professionalism: A study of high school teachers. U.S. Office of Education, Cooperative Research Project No. 330, 1962. (A revised version of the author's Ph.D. dissertation by the same title, University of Michigan, 1961.)

Colombotos, J. Sex role and professionalism: A study of high school teachers. *School Review* 71:27–40, 1963.

Colombotos, J. Physicians' attitudes toward Medicare. *Medical Care* 6:320–331, 1968.

Colombotos, J. Personal versus telephone interviews: Effect on responses. *Public Health Reports* 84:773–782, 1969a.

Colombotos, J. Physicians' attitudes toward a county health department: Ideology and self-interest. *Am. J. Public Health* 59:53–59, 1969b.

Colombotos, J. Physicians and Medicare; A before-after study of the effects of legislation on attitudes. *Am. Sociol. Rev.* 34:318–334, 1969c.

Colombotos, J. Social origins and ideology of physicians: A study of the effects of early socialization. *J. Health and Social Behavior* 10:16–29, 1969d.

Colombotos, J. Doctors' responses to new programs in medical care: Some projections. *Inquiry* 8:20–26, 1971.

Colombotos, J., Charles, C. A., and Kirchner, C. Physicians' attitudes toward political and health care policy issues in cross-national perspective: A comparison of FMGs and USMGs. *Social Science & Med.* 11:603–609, 1977.

Colombotos, J., and Indyk, D. Geriatrics as an emerging specialty: A commentary. Paper presented at the Annual Meeting of the American Public Health Association, Nov. 15, 1983.

Colombotos, J., and Kirchner, C. Physicians' perceptions and attitudes toward national health insurance: A case study of "anticipatory fait accompli" and "pluralistic ignorance." Proceedings, Annual Meeting of the American Statistics Association, Social Statistics Section, August 13, 1979, Washington, D.C.

Colombotos, J., Kirchner, C., and Millman, M. Doctors' attitudes toward peer reviews: A national study. Paper presented at the annual meeting of the Conference on Social Sciences in Health, American Public Health Association, 1975a.

Colombotos, J., Kirchner, C., and Millman, M. Physicians view national health insurance: A national study. *Medical Care* 13:369-396, 1975b.

Colombotos, J., Kirchner, C., and Millman, M. Promoting the policy-relevance of a study of physicians' attitudes toward health care issues. New York: Columbia University, March 30, 1976.

Committee on the Costs of Medical Care. *Medical Care for the American People.* Chicago: University of Chicago Press, 1932.

Congressional Budget Office. *Controlling Rising Hospital Costs.* Washington, DC: U.S. Government Printing Office, 1979.

Congressional Budget Office. *The Impact of PSRO's on Health Care Costs: An Update of CBO's 1979 Evaluation.* Washington, DC: U.S. Government Printing Office, 1981.

Congressional Budget Office. *Containing Medical Costs Through Market Forces.* Washington, DC: U.S. Government Printing Office, 1982.

Converse, P. E. The nature of belief systems in mass publics. In Apter, D. E. (Ed.), *Ideology and Discontent.* New York: Free Press, 1964, pp. 206-261.

Converse, P. E. *The Dynamics of Party Support: Cohort-analyzing Party Identification.* Beverly Hills, CA: Sage Publications, 1976.

Coser, R. L. Authority and decision-making in a hospital. *Am. Sociol. Rev.* 23:56-64, 1958.

Davis, J. A. *Undergraduate Career Decisions.* Chicago: Aldine, 1965.

Davis, K., Gold, M., and Makuc, D. Access to health care for the poor: Does the gap remain? *Annual Rev. Public Health* 2:159-182, 1981.

Davis, K., and Schoen, C. *Health and the War on Poverty: A Ten Year Appraisal.* Washington, DC: The Brookings Institution, 1978.

Demkovich, L. Urban voluntary hospitals caught in price squeeze face bleak future. *National J.,* pp. 1131-1136, 1982.

Derbyshire, R. *Medical Licensure and Discipline in the U.S.* Baltimore: Johns Hopkins Press, 1969.

Deuschle, J. M., Alvarez, B., Logsdon, D. N., Stahl, W. M., and Smith, H., Jr. Physician performance in a prepaid health plan: Results of the peer review program of the Health Insurance Plan of Greater New York. *Medical Care* 20:127-142, 1982.

Deutsch, M., and Collins, M. E. *Interracial Housing: A Psychological Evaluation of a Social Experiment.* Minneapolis: University of Minnesota Press, 1951.

Deutscher, I. Words and deeds. *Social Problems* 13:235-254, 1966.

Dibble, V. Occupations and ideologies. *Am. J. Sociol.* 68:229-241, 1962.

Dicey, A. V. *Law and Opinion in England during the Nineteenth Century.* Second Edition. London: Macmillan, 1914.

Donabedian, A. An evaluation of prepaid group practice. *Inquiry* 6:3-27, 1969.

Dowling, M. J. Directions for social policy analysis development: The sobering 80's. *Administration in Social Work* 6:73-89, 1982.

Ducker, D. G. The Effects of Two Sources of Role Strain on Women Physicians. Ph.D. Dissertation, City University of New York, 1974.

Durkheim, E. *Professional Ethics and Civic Morals.* Westport, CT: Greenwood Press, 1957.

Dutton, D. B. Explaining the low use of health services by the poor: Costs, attitudes or delivery systems. *Am. Sociol. Rev.* 43:348-368, 1978.

Eckstein, H. *Pressure Group Politics: The Case of the British Medical Association.* Stanford, CA: Stanford University Press, 1960.

Editorial, *J. Am. Med. Assoc.,* p. 1950, Dec. 3, 1932.

Editorial. *N.Y.S. J. Med.* 65:2779, 1965.

Ehrenreich, B., and Ehrenreich, J. The professional-managerial class. *Radical America* 11:7-31, 1977.

Eisenberg, J. M. Physician utilization: The state of research about physicians' practice patterns. *Medical Care* 23:461–483, 1985.

Eisenberg, J. M., Kitz, D. S., and Webber, R. A. Development of attitudes about sharing decision-making: A comparison of medical and surgical residents. *J. Health & Social Behavior* 24:85–90, 1983.

Elder, G. H., Jr. Age differentiation and the life course. In Inkeles, A., Coleman, J., and Smelser, N. (Eds.), *Annual Review of Sociology.* Palo Alto: Annual Reviews, 1975, pp. 165–190.

Elder, G. H., Jr. Adolescence in historical perspective. In Adelson, J. (Ed.), *Handbook of Adolescent Psychology.* New York: Wiley, 1980, pp. 3–46.

Elinson, J. Discussion of papers presented at the session, 'Have we narrowed the gaps in health status between the poor and nonpoor'? *Medical Care* 15(8):675–678, 1977.

Elinson, J., and Siegmann, A. E. (Eds.). *Sociomedical Health Indicators.* New York: Baywood, 1977.

Emerson, R. M. Social exchange theory. In Rosenberg, M. and Turner, R. H. (Eds.), *Social Psychology: Sociological Perspectives.* New York: Basic Books, 1981, pp. 30–65.

Enthoven, A. C. *Health Plan: The Only Practical Solution to the Soaring Cost of Health Care.* Menlo Park, CA: Addison-Wesley, 1980.

Eron, L. The effect of medical education on attitudes: A follow-up study. In Gee, H. H. and Glaser, R. J. (Eds.), *The Ecology of the Medical Student.* Evanston, IL: Association of American Medical Colleges, 1958, pp. 25–33.

Erskine, H. The polls: Health insurance. *Public Opinion Q.* 39:128–143, 1975.

Etzioni, A. Epilogue: Alternative conceptions of accountability. In Greenfield, H. I. (Ed.), *Accountability in Health Facilities.* New York: Praeger, 1975, pp. 121–142.

Evan, W. M. Law as an instrument of social change. In Gouldner, A. W. and Miller, S. M. (Eds.), *Applied Sociology.* New York: Free Press, 1965, pp. 285–293.

Farnsworth, D. L. Annual discourse—youth in protest. *N. Engl. J. Med.* 282:1235–1240, 1970.

Feingold, E. *Medicare: Policy and Politics.* San Francisco: Chandler, 1966.

Feldstein, P. J. *Health Associations and the Demand for Legislation.* Cambridge, MA: Ballinger, 1977.

Fink, R. HMO physician recruitment stymied by higher fee-for-service salaries. *Group Health News* 21:8, 1980.

Foster, M. Attitudes of Canadian Physicians in the United States: The Role of Selection and Socialization. Ph.D. Dissertation, Columbia University, 1976.

Fox, R. Physicians on the drug industry side of the prescription blank: Their dual commitment to medical science and business. *J. Health and Hum. Behavior* 2:3–16, 1961.

Fox, R. Is there a 'new' medical student. *Ethics of Health Care.* Washington, DC: National Academy of Sciences, 1974, pp. 197–220.

Fox, R. The medicalization and demedicalization of American society. *Daedalus* 106:9–22, 1977.

Freidson, E. Client control and medical practice. *Am. J. Sociol.* 65:374–382, 1960.

Freidson, E. *Patients' Views of Medical Practice.* New York: Russell Sage, 1961.

Freidson, E. *Profession of Medicine.* New York: Dodd, Mead, 1970.

Freidson, E. *Doctoring Together: A Study of Professional Social Control.* New York: Elsevier, 1975.

Freidson, E. The organization of medical practice. In Freeman, H. E., Levine, B., and Reeder, L. G. (Eds.), *Handbook of Medical Sociology,* Third Edition. Englewood Cliffs, NJ: Prentice-Hall, 1979, pp. 297–307.

Freymann, J. G. Leadership in American medicine: A matter of personal responsibility. *N. Engl. J. Med.* 270:710-720, 1964.

Fuchs, L. H. Sources of Jewish internationalism and liberalism. In Sklare, M. (Ed.), *The Jews.* Glencoe, IL: Free Press, 1958, pp. 595-613.

Fuchs, V. R. *Who Shall Live?* New York: Basic Books, 1974.

Fuchs, V. R. Sounding board: The coming challenge to American physicians. *N. Engl. J. Med.* 304(24):1487-1490, 1981.

The Fuller Utilization of the Woman Physician. Report on a conference on Meeting Medical Manpower Needs. Women's Bureau, U.S. Department of Labor, Washington, DC, Jan. 12-13, 1968.

Funkenstein, D. H. *Medical Students, Medical Schools, and Society During Five Eras: Factors Affecting the Career Choices of Physicians, 1958-1976.* Cambridge, MA: Ballinger, 1978.

Gaffin, B. and Associates. *What Americans Think of the Medical Profession: Report on a Public Opinion Study.* Chicago: American Medical Association, 1956.

Gapen, P. Minority admissions: The increasingly empty promise of affirmative action. *The New Physician* 28:20-24, 1979.

Garceau, O. *The Political Life of the American Medical Association.* Hamden, CT: Archon Books, 1941.

Gecas, V. The influence of social class in socialization. In Burr, W. R., Hill, R., Nye, F. I., and Reiss, I. L. (Eds.), *Contemporary Themes About the Family.* Vol. 1. New York: Free Press, 1979, pp. 127-161.

Gecas, V. Contexts of socialization. In Rosenberg, M. and Turner, R. L. (Eds.), *Social Psychology: Sociological Perspectives.* New York: Basic Books, 1981, pp. 165-199.

Gee, H. H., and Glaser, R. J. (Eds.). *The Ecology of the Medical Student.* Evanston, IL: Association of American Medical Colleges, 1958.

Ginzberg, E. Procompetition in health care: Policy or fantasy. *Milbank Memorial Fund Q./ Health and Society* 60:386-398, 1981.

Ginzberg, E. Allied health resources. In Mechanic, D. (Ed.), *Handbook of Health, Health Care, and the Health Professions.* New York: Free Press, 1983a, pp. 479-494.

Ginzberg, E. How many physicians are enough? *Ann. Am. Acad. of Political and Social Sciences* 468:205-215, 1983b.

Ginzberg, E., Brann, E., Hiestand, D., and Ostow, M. The expanding physician supply and health policy: The clouded outlook. *Milbank Memorial Fund Q./Health & Society* 59(4):508-541, 1981.

Glaser, W. A. Doctors and politics. *Am. J. Sociol.* 66:230-245, 1960.

Glazer, N. The social policy of the Reagan administration: A review. *The Public Interest* 75:76-98, 1984.

Glazer, N., and Moynihan, D. P. *Beyond the Melting Pot.* Cambridge, MA: M.I.T. Press, 1963.

Glenn, N. D. *Cohort Analysis.* Beverly Hills, CA: Sage Publications, 1977.

Glenn, N. D., and Hill, L., Jr. Rural-urban differences in attitudes and behavior in the United States. *Ann. Am. Acad. of Political and Social Sciences* 429:36-50, 1977.

Glenn, N. D., and Simmons, J. L. Are regional cultural differences diminishing? *Public Opinion Q.* 31:176-193, 1967.

Goldman, L. Doctors' attitudes toward national health insurance. *Medical Care* 12:413-423, 1974a.

Goldman, L. Factors related to physicians' medical and political attitudes: A documentation of intraprofessional variations. *J. Health and Social Behavior* 15:177-187, 1974b.

Goldman, L., and Ebbert, A., Jr. The fate of medical student liberalism: A prediction. *J. Med. Educ.* 48:1095–1103, 1973.

Goldsmith, J. C. Competition: How will it affect hospitals? *Health Care Financial Management*, p. 16, Nov. 1981.

Goode, W. J. Community within a community: The professions. *Am. Sociol. Rev.* 22:194–200, 1957.

Goodman, L. J., and Steiber, S. R. Public support for national health insurance. *Am. J. Public Health* 71:1105–1108, 1981.

Goslin, D. A. (Ed.). *Handbook of Socialization Theory and Research.* Chicago: Rand McNally, 1969.

Goss, M. E. W. Influence and authority among physicians in an outpatient clinic. *Am. Sociol. Rev.* 26:39–50, 1961.

Gouldner, A. W. Cosmopolitans and locals: Toward an analysis of latent social roles—I and II. *Admin. Science Q.* 2(Dec.):281–306, 1957; (Mar.):444–480, 1958.

Gray, B. H. An introduction to the new health care for profit. In Gray, B. H. (Ed.), *The New Health Care for Profit.* Washington: National Academy Press, 1983, pp. 1–16.

Gray, R. M., Newman, W. R. E., and Reinhardt, A. M. The effect of medical specialization on physicians' attitudes. *J. Health and Hum. Behavior* 7:128–132, 1966.

Greeley, A. M. *Religion and Career: A Study of College Graduates.* New York: Sheed and Ward, 1963.

Green, M. The gang that can't deregulate. *The New Republic*, pp. 14–17, 1983.

Grenell, B. Correlates of Specialty Choice of Female Medical Students. Ph.D. Dissertation, Columbia University, 1979.

Gritzer, G. Division of Labor in Medicine: The Case of Rehabilitation. Ph.D. Dissertation, New York University, 1978.

Gross, N., Mason, W., and McEachern, A. *Explorations in Role Analysis: Studies of the School Superintendent Role.* New York: Wiley, 1958.

Hall, O. The informal organization of the medical profession. *Canadian J. Economics & Political Science* 44:30–44, 1946.

Hall, O. The stages of a medical career. *Am. J. Sociol.* 53:327–336, 1948.

Halpern, S. A. Segmental Professionalization within Medicine: The Case of Pediatrics. Ph.D. Dissertation, University of California, 1982.

Hamilton, R. F., and Wright, J. *New Directions in Political Sociology.* Indianapolis: Bobbs-Merrill, 1975.

Hanft, R. S. Health manpower. In Jonas, S. (Ed.), *Health Care Delivery in the U.S.* Second Edition. New York: Springer, 1981, pp. 61–95.

Harris, R. *A Sacred Trust.* New York: New American Library, 1966.

Havighurst, C. C. *Deregulating the Health Care Industry: Planning for Competition.* Cambridge, MA: Ballinger, 1982.

Havighurst, R. J., and Neugarten, B. L. *Society and Education.* Third Edition. Boston: Allyn and Bacon, 1967.

Health Information Foundation. Where physicians work. *Progress in Health Services* 13, University of Chicago, 1964.

Heberle, R. *Social Movements.* New York: Appleton-Century-Crofts, 1951.

Heins, M. Career and life patterns of women and men physicians. In Shapiro, E. C., and Loewenstein, L. M. (Eds.), *Becoming a Physician.* Cambridge, MA: Ballinger, 1979, pp. 217–236.

Held, P. J., and Reinhardt, U. E. Prepaid medical practice: A summary of findings from a recent survey of group practices in the United States. *Group Health J.* 1:4–15, Summer 1980.

Hill, R. J. Attitudes and behavior. In Rosenberg, M. and Turner, R. H. (Eds.), *Social Psychology: Sociological Perspectives*. New York: Basic Books, 1981, pp. 347–377.

Hovland, C. I., Lumsdaine, A. A., and Sheffield, F. D. *Experiments on Mass Communication, Vol. III, Studies in Social Psychology in World War II*. Princeton: Princeton University Press, 1949.

Howard, J., and Strauss, A. (Eds.). *Humanizing Health Care*. New York: Wiley, 1975.

Hudson, R. B., and Binstock, R. H. Political systems and aging. In Binstock, R. H. and Shanas, E. (Eds.), *Handbook of Aging and the Social Sciences*. New York: Van Nostrand Reinhold, 1976, pp. 369–400.

Hughes, E. C. Dilemmas and contradictions of status. *Am. J. Sociol.* 50:353–359, 1945.

Hughes, E. C. The making of a physician. *Human Organization* 14:21–25, 1955.

Hughes, E. C. *The Sociological Eye*. Vol. 2. New York: Atherton, 1971.

Hughes, E. C., MacGill-Hughes, H., and Deutscher, I. *Twenty Thousand Nurses Tell Their Story*. Philadelphia: Lippincott, 1958.

Hyman, H. *Interviewing in Social Research*. Chicago: University of Chicago Press, 1954.

Hyman, H. *Survey Design and Analysis*. Glencoe, IL: Free Press, 1955.

Hyman, H., *Political Socialization*. Glencoe, IL: Free Press, 1959.

Hyman, H., and Sheatsley, P. B. Attitudes toward desegregation. *Scientific American* 211:3, 1964.

Iglehart, J. Health policy report: Federal policies and the poor. *N. Engl. J. Med.* 307;836–840, 1982a.

Iglehart, J. Will Medicare's success spoil its chance to survive spending cuts? *National J.*, pp. 772–775, 1982b.

Iglehart, J. HMO's (for-profit and not-for-profit) on the move. *N. Engl. J. Med.* 310(18):1203–1208, 1984.

The Insider's Newsletter. New York, February 8, 1965.

Interest groups pressing for earlier, more active role in electoral process. *National J.* pp. 1005–1010, 1983.

Janowitz, M. *The Professional Soldier*. Glencoe, IL: Free Press, 1960.

Jeffe, D., and Jeffe, S. B. Losing patience with doctors: Physicians vs. the public on health care costs. *Public Opinion*, pp. 45–55, Feb./Mar. 1984.

Johnson, T. J. *Professions and Power*. London: Macmillan, 1972.

Johnstone, J. W. C., Slawski, E. J., and Bowman, W. W. *The News People*. Urbana, IL: University of Illinois Press, 1976.

Jonas, S. *Health Care Delivery in the United States*. Second Edition. New York: Springer, 1981.

Jonas, S., and Banta, D. Government in the health care system. In Jonas, S. (Ed.), *Health Care Delivery in the United States*. Second Edition. New York: Springer, 1981, pp. 313–351.

Kandel, D. B. The Career Decisions of Medical Students: A Study of Occupational Recruitment and Occupational Choice. Ph.D. Dissertation, Columbia University, 1960.

Kandel, D. B. Drug and drinking behavior among youth. In Inkeles, A., Smelser, N. J., and Turner, R. H. (Eds.), *Annual Review of Sociology*. Palo Alto: Annual Reviews, 1980, pp. 235–285.

Kanter, M. *Men and Women of the Corporation*. New York: Basic Books, 1977.

Katz, D. The functional approach to the study of attitudes. *Public Opinion Q.* 24:163–204, 1960.

Kehrer, B. H. Factors influencing the incomes of men and women physicians. *J. Human Resources* 11:526–545, 1976.

Kendall, P. L. The relationship between medical educators and medical practitioners:

Sources of strain and occasions for cooperation. *J. Med. Educ.* 40:1, Part 2:137–245, 1965.

Kendall, P. L. Medical specialization: Trends and contributing factors, consequences of the trend toward specialization. In Coombs, R. H. and Vincent, C. E. (Eds.), *Psychosocial Aspects of Medical Training.* Springfield, IL: Thomas, 1971, pp. 449–497.

Kendall, P. L. Theory and research: The case of studies in medical education. In Coser, L. A. (Ed.), *The Idea of Social Structure: Papers in Honor of Robert K. Merton.* New York: Harcourt Brace Jovanovich, 1975, pp. 301–321.

Kendall, P. L., and Selvin, H. C. Tendencies toward specialization in medical training. In Merton, R. K., Reader, G. G., and Kendall, P. L. (Eds.), *The Student Physician.* Cambridge, MA: Harvard University Press, 1957, pp. 153–174.

Kertzer, D. Generation as a sociological problem. In Turner, R. and Short, J. F., Jr. (Eds.), *Annual Review of Sociology.* Palto Alto: Annual Reviews, 1983, pp. 125–149.

Killian, L. M. The Negro in American Society. *Florida State University Studies* 28:65–70, 1958.

Klein, R. The politics of ideology vs. the reality of politics: The case of Britain's National Health Service in the 1980s. *Milbank Memorial Fund Q. Health and Society* 62:82–109, 1984.

Knapp, R. H., and Goodrich, H. B. *Origins of American Scientists.* Chicago: University of Chicago Press, 1952.

Knoke, D. *Change and Continuity in American Politics.* Baltimore: Johns Hopkins University Press, 1976.

Knowles, J. (Ed.). *Doing Better and Feeling Worse: Health in the U.S. Daedalus* 106(1), 1977.

Kohn, M. L., and Schooler, C. *Work and Personality: An Inquiry into the Impact of Social Stratification.* Norwood, NJ: Ablex Publishing Co., 1983.

Kuhn, T. S. *The Structure of Scientific Revolutions.* Second Edition. Chicago: University of Chicago Press, 1970.

Kutner, B., Wilkins, C., and Yarrow, P. R. Verbal attitudes and overt behavior involving racial prejudice. *J. Abnormal & Social Psychology* 47:649–652, 1952.

Ladd, E. C. Public opinion questions at the quinquennial. *Public Opinion,* pp. 20–41, April/May 1983.

Ladd, E. C., and Hadley, C. D. *Transformations of the American Party System.* New York: Norton, 1978.

Ladd, E. C., and Lipset, S. M. *The Divided Academy: Professors and Politics.* New York: McGraw-Hill, 1975.

Ladinsky, J. Careers of lawyers, law practice, and legal institutions. *Am. Sociol. Rev.* 28:47–54, 1963.

Lally, J. Selection as an interactive process: The case of Catholic psychoanalysts and psychiatrists. *Social Science & Med.* 9:157–164, 1975.

LaPiere, R. T. Attitudes vs. actions. *Social Forces* 13:230–237, 1934.

Larson, M. L. *The Rise of Professionalism: A Sociological Analysis.* Berkeley, CA: University of California Press, 1977.

Lazarsfeld, P. F. Mutual effects of statistical variables. Bureau of Applied Social Research, Columbia University, 1947. (Mimeo.)

Lazarsfeld, P. F. Mutual relations over time of two attributes: A review and integration of various approaches. Columbia University, 1971. (Mimeo.)

Lazarsfeld, P. F. Some episodes in the history of panel analysis. In Kandel, D. B. (Ed.), *Longitudinal Research on Drug Use.* New York: Wiley, 1978, pp. 249–265.

Lazarsfeld, P. F., Berelson, B., and Gaudet, H. *The People's Choice*. Second Edition. Chicago: University of Chicago Press, 1948.

Lee, P. R., and Estes, C. L. New federalism and health policy. *Ann. Am. Acad. of Political and Social Sciences* 468:87–102, 1983.

Lenski, G. *The Religious Factor*. Garden City, NY: Doubleday, 1961.

Lerner, M., and Stutz, R. N. Have we narrowed the gaps between the poor and non-poor? Part II. Narrowing the gaps, 1959–1961 to 1969–1971: Mortality. *Medical Care* 15(8):620–635, 1977.

Leserman, J. Changes in the professional orientation of medical students: A follow-up study. *J. Med. Educ.* 55:415–422, 1980.

Levinson, D. J. Medical education and the theory of adult socialization. *J. Health and Social Behavior* 8:253–265, 1967.

Levinson, D. *The Seasons of a Man's Life*. New York: Knopf, 1978.

Levy, L. Factors which facilitate or impede transfer of medical functions from physicians to paramedical personnel. *J. Health & Human Behavior* 7(1):50–54, 1966.

Lewis, C. E. Students, social change, and community health. *Arch. Environ. Health* 18:67–71, 1969a.

Lewis, C. E. A longitudinal study of potential change agents in medicine—a preliminary report. *J. Med. Educ.* 44:1029–1034, 1969b.

Lewis, C. E., and Winer, S. Has idealism survived? *The New Physician* 25:24–29, 1976.

Light, D. W. Medical and nursing education: Surface behavior and deep structure. In Mechanic, D. (Ed.), *Handbook of Health, Health Care, and the Health Professions*, New York: Free Press, 1983, pp. 455–478.

Lipset, S. M. *Political Man: The Social Bases of Politics*. Garden City, NY: Doubleday, Anchor Books edition, 1963. (Originally published by Doubleday, 1960.)

Lipset, S. M. *Revolution and Counter-Revolution: Change and Persistence in Social Structures*. New York: Anchor Books, 1970.

Lipset, S. M., and Bendix, R. *Social Mobility in Industrial Society*. Berkeley: University of California Press, 1964.

Lipset, S. M., and Schwartz, M. A. The politics of professionals. In Vollmer, H. M. and Mills, D. L. (Eds.), *Professionalization*. Englewood Cliffs, NJ: Prentice-Hall, 1966, pp. 299–310.

Lipset, S. M., Trow, M., and Coleman, J. *Union Democracy: The Inside Politics of the International Typographical Union*. Glencoe, IL: Free Press, 1956.

Litwak, E. Models of bureaucracy which permit conflict. *Am. J. Sociol.* 67:177–184, 1961.

Long, S. H., Settle, R. F., and Link, C. R. Who has the burden of Medicare cost sharing? *Inquiry* 19:222–234, 1982.

Lorber, J. *Women Physicians: Careers, Status, and Power*. New York: Methuen, 1984.

Louis Harris and Associates. *Medical Practice in the 1980's: Physicians' Look at Their Changing Profession*, New York, 1981.

Louis Harris and Associates. *The Equitable Healthcare Survey: Options for Controlling Costs*. (A survey of the American Public and Selected Professionals in the Health Care Field.) New York, 1983.

Louis Harris and Associates. *The Equitable Healthcare Survey II: Physicians' Attitudes toward Cost Containment*, New York, 1984.

Lublin, J. S., and Conte, C. Federal de-regulation runs into a backlash even from business. *The Wall Street J.*, p. 1, Dec. 14, 1983.

Luft, H. S. Economic incentives and clinical decisions. In Gray, B. H. (Ed.), *The New Health Care for Profit*. Washington: National Academy Press, 1983, pp. 103–123.

Lyden, F. J., Geiger, H. J., and Peterson, O. L. *The Training of Good Physicians: Critical Factors in Career Choices.* Cambridge, MA: Harvard University Press, 1968.

Maccoby, E. E. Pitfalls in the analysis of panel data: A research note on some technical aspects of *Voting. Am. J. Sociol.* 61:359-362, 1956.

Maccoby, E. E., Matthews, R. E., and Morton, A. S. Youth and political change. *Public Opinion Q.* 18:23-39, 1954.

MacColl, W. A. *Group Practice and Prepayment of Medical Care.* Washington: Public Affairs Press, 1966.

MacIver, R. M. *The More Perfect Union.* New York: Macmillan, 1948.

MacIver, R. M. *Foreword.* In Berger, M., *Equality by Statute.* New York: Columbia University Press, 1954.

Mayhew, L. H. *Law and Equal Opportunity.* Cambridge, MA: Harvard University Press, 1968.

Mannheim, K. The problem of generations. In *Essays on the Sociology of Knowledge.* London: Routledge and Kegan Paul, 1952, pp. 276-322.

Margolis, R. J. National health insurance—The dream whose time has come? In Conrad, P. and Kern, R. (Eds.), *The Sociology of Health and Illness: Critical Perspectives.* New York: St. Martin's Press, 1981, pp. 486-501.

Marmor, T. R., and Dunham, A. The politics of health. In Mechanic, D. (Ed.), *The Handbook of Health, Health Care and the Health Professions.* New York: Free Press, 1983, pp. 67-80.

Mason, K. O., Mason, W. M., Winsborough, H. H., and Poole, W. K. Some methodological issues in cohort analysis of archival data. *Am. Sociol. Rev.* 38:242-258, 1973.

McCandless, B. R. Childhood socialization. In Goslin, D. A., *Handbook of Socialization Theory and Research.* Chicago: Rand McNally, 1969, pp. 791-820.

McClosky, H., Hoffman, P. J., and O'Hara, R. Issue conflict and consensus among party leaders and followers. *Am. Political Science Rev.* 54:406-427, 1960.

McDermott, W. Medicine: The public's good and one's own. *World Health Forum* 1(1,2):123-131, 1980.

McGarvey, M. D., Mullan, F., and Sharfstein, S. S. A study in medical action—The Student Health Organizations. *N. Engl. J. Med.* 279:74-80, 1968.

McGuire, W. J. A syllogistic analysis of cognitive relationships. In Rosenberg, M. J., Hovland, C. I., McGuire, W. J., and Brehm, J. W. (Eds.), *Attitude Organization and Change: An Analysis of Consistency Among Attitude Components.* New Haven: Yale University Press, 1960, pp. 65-111.

McGuire, W. J. The nature of attitudes and attitude change. In Lindzey, G. and Aronson, E. (Eds.), *Handbook of Social Psychology,* Vol. 3. Reading, MA: Addison-Wesley, 1969. pp. 136-314.

McKinlay, J. B. On the professional regulation of change. In Halmos, P. (Ed.), *Professionalization and Social Change.* Keele: Keele University, 1973, pp. 61-84.

Means, J. *Doctors, People, and Government.* Boston: Little, Brown, 1953.

Mechanic, D. Human problems and the organization of health care. *Ann. Am. Acad. of Political and Social Sciences* 399:1-11, 1972.

Mechanic, D. Factors affecting receptivity to innovations in health care delivery among primary-care physicians. In Mechanic, D. (Ed.), *Politics, Medicine, and Social Science.* New York: Wiley, 1974, pp. 69-87.

Medical education in the United States, 1972-73, *J. Amer. Med. Assoc.* 226:902, 1973.

Medical education in the United States, 1975-76, *J. Am. Med. Assoc.* 236:2962, 1976.

Medical education in the United States, 1982-83. *J. Am. Med. Assoc.* 250:1513, 1983.

Medical students: Healers become activists. *Saturday Rev.,* pp. 41-54, Aug. 16, 1969.

Medical Tribune, 2:1, May 15, 1961.

Medicine's own generation gap. *Med. World News* 10:23–30, June 6, 1969.

Meltsner, A. J. Political feasibility and policy analysis. *Public Administration Review* 32:859–867, 1972.

Merton, R. K. *Social Theory and Social Structure*. Revised Edition. Glencoe, IL: Free Press, 1957.

Merton, R. K., Bloom, S., and Ramsöy, N. R. Studies in the sociology of medical education. *J. Med. Educ.* 31:552–565, 1956.

Merton, R. K., Reader, G. G. and Kendall, P. L. (Eds.). *The Student Physician*. Cambridge: Harvard University Press, 1957.

Michels, R. *Political Parties*. New York: Hearst's International Library, 1915.

Mick, S. S., and Worobey, J. L. Foreign medical graduates in the 1980's: Trends in specialization. *Am. J. Public Health* 74:698–703, 1984.

Mihalski, E. J. The new era of utilization and quality control: Professional Review Organizations. *Bull. NY Acad. Med.* 60(1):48–53, 1984.

Milio, N. *The Case of Health in Communities: Access for Outcasts*. New York: Macmillan, 1975.

Mooney, A. The great society and health: Policies for narrowing the gaps in health status between the poor and non-poor. *Medical Care* 15(8):611–619, 1977.

Moore, W. E. Occupational socialization. In Goslin, D. A. (Ed.), *Handbook of Socialization Theory and Research*. Chicago: Rand McNally, 1969, pp. 861–883.

Moore, W. E. *The Professions: Roles and Rules*. New York: Russell Sage Foundation, 1970.

"Morris Fishbein, M.D." *N. Engl. J. Med.* 295:1134–1135, 1976.

Mortimer, J. T., and Simmons, R. G. Adult socialization. In Turner, R. H., Coleman, J., and Fox, R. C. (Eds.), *Annual Review of Sociology*. Palo Alto: Annual Reviews, 1978, pp. 421–454.

Muir, W. K. *Prayer in the Public Schools: Law and Attitude Change*. Chicago: University of Chicago Press, 1967.

Mussen, P. H. Some personality and social factors related to changes in children's attitudes toward Negroes. *J. Abnormal & Social Psychol.* 45:423–441, 1950.

Myrdal, G. *An American Dilemma*. New York: Harper and Row, 1944.

National Opinion Research Center. *Basic Tabulations, 1955 Health Attitude Study: Doctor Questionnaire*, undated.

National Opinion Research Center. *General Social Surveys, 1972–80: Cumulative Codebook*. Chicago, July 1980.

Navarro, V. Where is the popular mandate? A reply to the conventional wisdom. *Int. J. Health Services* 13:169–174, 1983.

Navarro, V. *Medicine Under Capitalism*. New York: Prodist, 1976.

The new doctor, community practice and the money barrier. *Medical Dimensions* 1:4–5, 46, April, 1972.

Newcomb, T. M. An approach to the study of communicative acts. *Psychol. Bull.* 60:393–404, 1953.

Nie, N. H., Hull, C. H., Jenkins, J. G., Steinbrenner, K., and Bent, D. H. *Statistical Package for the Social Sciences*. Second Edition. New York: McGraw-Hill, 1975.

Numbers, R. L. *Almost Persuaded: American Physicians and Compulsory Health Insurance, 1912–1920*. Baltimore: Johns Hopkins University Press, 1978.

Nunnally, J. C. *Psychometric Theory*. New York: McGraw-Hill, 1967.

Office of Technology Assessment. *Strategies for Medical Technology Assessment*. Washington, DC: U.S. Government Printing Office, 1982.

O'Gorman, H. Pluralistic ignorance and white estimates of white support for racial segregation. *Public Opinion Q.* 39:311–330, 1975.

Olesen, V. L., and Whittaker, E. W. *The Silent Dialogue.* San Francisco: Jossey-Bass, 1968.

Olson, M. (Ed.). *A New Approach to the Economics of Health Care.* Washington, DC: American Enterprise Institute, 1982.

Otis, G. D., Quenk, N., Weiss, J., Albert, M., Offir, J., and Richardson, C. *Medical Specialty Selection: A Review and Bibliography Report for the U.S.-DHEW Bureau of Health Resources Development.* Washington, DC: U.S. Government Printing Office, DHEW Publication No. (HRA)75-8, 1974.

Parental income of 1981 first-year medical school applicants and accepted students. *J. Med. Educ.* 58:829–830, 1983.

Parsons, T. Social change and medical organization in the United States: A sociological perspective. *Ann. Am. Acad. of Political and Social Sciences* 346:21–33, 1963.

Pastore, N. *The Nature-Nurture Conflict.* New York: Kings Crown Press, 1948.

Pear, R. Nursing homes offer strong argument for de-regulation. *N.Y. Times,* Oct. 23, 1983.

Pelz, D. C., and Andrews, F. M. Detecting causal priorities in panel study data. *Am. Sociol. Rev.* 29:836–848, 1964.

Phillips, R. R., and Dorsey, J. L. A look inside: Some aspects of structure and function in forty group practice HMO's. *Group Health J.* 1:16–32, Summer 1980.

Physicians Forum. *The Salaried Physician.* New York, 1982.

Pound, R. *The Task of Law.* Lancaster, PA: Franklin and Marshall College, 1944.

Rayack, E. *Professional Power and American Medicine; the Economics of the American Medical Association.* Cleveland: World, 1967.

Reader, G. G. Development of professional attitudes and capacities. In Gee, H. H. and Glaser, R. J. (Eds), *The Ecology of the Medical Student.* Evanston, IL: Association of American Medical Colleges, 1958, pp. 164–185.

Redman, E. *The Dance of Legislation.* New York: Simon and Schuster, 1973.

Reilly, B. J., and Legge, S. L. The embattled hospital: Cost containment vs. imperatives for expansion. *J. Health Politics, Policy and Law* 7:254–270, 1982.

Reinhardt, U. W. Table manners at the health care feast. In Yaggy, D. and Anylan, W. G. (Eds.), *Financing Health Care: Competition vs. Regulation.* Cambridge, MA: Ballinger, 1982.

Relman, A. The new medical industrial complex. *N. Engl. J. Med.* 303:963–970, 1980.

Renshon, S. A. *Handbook of Political Socialization.* New York: Free Press, 1977.

Ricardo-Campbell, R. *The Economics and Politics of Health.* Chapel Hill: University of North Carolina Press, 1982.

Richard, M. P. The Negro physician: Babbitt or revolutionary? *J. Health and Social Behavior* 10:265–274, Dec. 1969.

Riley, M. W., Johnson, M. J., and Foner, A. *Aging and Society, Vol. 3: A Sociology of Age Stratification.* New York: Russell Sage Foundation, 1972.

Rivlin, A. M. *Systematic Thinking for Social Action.* Washington, DC: The Brookings Institute, 1971.

Robinson, J. The ups and downs and ins and outs of ideology. *Public Opinion,* pp. 12–15, Feb./Mar. 1984.

Roche, J. P., and Gordon, M. M. Can morality be legislated. In Young, K. and Mack, R. W. (Eds.), *Principles of Sociology: A Reader in Theory and Research.* New York: American Book, 1960, pp. 337–342.

Rodgers, W. L. Estimable functions of age, period, and cohort effects: Reply to comment by Smith, Mason, and Fienberg. *Am. Sociol. Rev.* 47:774–787: 793–796, 1982.

Roemer, M. I. Market failure and health care policy. *J. Public Health Policy* 3:419-431. 1982.

Rogers, T. *A Numerical Comparison of Five Indices of Mutual Effects.* New York: Bureau of Applied Social Research, Columbia University, 1967.

Rose, A. M. Sociological factors in the effectiveness of projected legislative remedies. *J. Legal Educ.* 11:470-481, 1959.

Rose, A. M. The passage of legislation: The politics of financing medical care for the aging. In Rose, A. M. (Ed.), *The Power Structure: Political Processes in American Society.* New York: Oxford University Press, 1967, pp. 400-455.

Rosen, G. *The Specialization of Medicine with Particular Reference to Ophthalmology.* New York: Froben Press, 1944.

Rosen, G. Some substantive limiting conditions in communication between health officers and medical practitioners. *Am. J. Public Health* 51:1805-1816, 1961.

Rosenberg, M. *Occupations and Values.* Glencoe, IL: Free Press, 1957.

Rosow, I. Forms and functions of adult socialization. *Social Forces* 44:35-45, 1965.

Rosow, I. *Socialization to Old Age.* Berkeley: University of California Press, 1974.

Rosten, L. C. *The Washington Correspondents.* New York: Harcourt, Brace, 1937.

Ryder, N. B. The cohort as a concept in the study of social change. *Am. Sociol. Rev.* 30:843-861, 1965.

Saenger, G., and Gilbert, E. Customer reactions to the integration of Negro sales personnel *Int. J. Opinion and Attitude Res.* 4:57-76, 1950.

Schattschneider, E. E. *The Semisovereign People.* Hinsdale, IL: Dryden Press, 1960.

Schiltz, M. E. *Public Attitudes Toward Social Security 1935-1965.* Research Report No. 33, Office of Research and Statistics, Social Security Administration. Washington, DC: U.S. Government Printing Office, 1970.

Schimel, D. Medicaid and Professional Standards Review Organizations. *Bull. NY Acad. Med.* 59(1):149-152, 1983.

Schroeder, S. A. National Health Insurance—always just around the corner. *Amer. J. Public Health* 71:1101-1103, 1981.

Schroeder, S. A., and Showstalk, J. A. The dynamics of medical technology use: Analysis and policy options. In Altman, S. H. and Blendon, R. (Eds.), *Medical Technology: The Culprit Behind Health Care Costs?* Proceedings of the 1977 Sun Valley Forum on National Health. Washington, DC: U.S. Government Printing Office, 1979.

Schwartz, M. A. *Trends in White Attitudes Toward Negroes.* Chicago: National Opinion Research Center, University of Chicago, 1967.

Schwartzbaum, A. M., and McGrath, J. H. The perception of prestige differences among medical subspecialties. *Social Science & Med.* 7:365-371, 1973.

Scott, J. F., and Scott, L. H. They are not so much anti-Negro as pro-middle class. *New York Times Magazine*, Mar. 24, 1968, pp. 46ff.

Scott, R. W. Professionals in bureaucracies: Areas of conflict. In Vollmer, H. M. and Mills, D. L. (Eds.), *Professionalization.* Englewood Cliffs, NJ: Prentice-Hall, 1966, pp. 265-276.

Seaman, M., and Evans, J. W. Stratification and hospital care. II. The objective criteria of performance. *Amer. Sociol. Rev.* 26:193-204, 1961.

Sears, D. O., Lau, R. R., Tyler, T. R., and Allen, H. M. Self-interest versus symbolic politics in policy attitudes and presidential voting. *Am. Political Science Rev.* 74:670-684, 1980.

A second look at last year's radicals. *Medical World News* 11:32-40, June 26, 1970.

Selvin, H. A critique of tests of statistical significance. *Amer. Sociol. Rev.* 22:519-527, 1957.

Sewell, W. H. Some recent developments in socialization theory and research. *Ann. Am. Acad. of Political Sciences* 349:163–181, 1963.

Shapiro, E. C., and Jones, A. B. Women physicians and the exercise of power and authority in health care. In Shapiro, E. C. and Loewenstein, L. M. (Eds.), *Becoming a Physician.* Cambridge, MA: Ballinger, 1979, pp. 237–245.

Sherlock, B. J., and Morris, R. T. *Becoming a Dentist.* Springfield, IL: Charles Thomas, 1971.

Shortell, S. M. Occupational prestige differences within the medical and allied health professions. *Social Science & Med.* 8:1–9, 1974.

Simpson, I. H. *From Student to Nurse: A Longitudinal Study of Socialization.* New York: Cambridge University Press, 1979.

Smith, H. L., Mason, W. M., and Fienberg, S. E. More chimeras of the age-period-cohort accounting framework: Comment on Rodgers. *Am. Sociol. Rev.* 47:787–793, 1982.

Somers, A. R. Moderating the rise in health costs: A pragmatic beginning. *N. Engl. J. Med.* 307:944–950, 1982.

Somers, H. M., and Somers, A. R. *Doctors, Patients, and Health Insurance.* Washington, D.C.: The Brookings Institution, 1961.

Somers, H. M., and Somers, A. R. *Medicare and the Hospitals: Issues and Prospects.* Washington, DC: The Brookings Institution, 1967.

Spivey, B. E. Are we physicians helpless? *N. Engl. J. Med.* 310(15):1116–1118, 1984.

Starr, P. The politics of therapeutic nihilism. *Hastings Center Report*, pp. 24–30, Oct. 1978.

Starr, P. *The Social Transformation of American Medicine.* New York: Basic Books, 1982.

Steiber, S. R., and Ferber, L. A. Support for national health insurance: Intercohort differentials. *Public Opinion Q.* 45:179–198, 1981.

Stern, B. J. *Society and Medical Progress.* Princeton: Princeton University Press, 1941.

Stevens, R. *American Medicine and the Public Interest.* New Haven: Yale University Press, 1971.

Stevens, R. Geriatric medicine in historical perspective: The pros and cons of geriatric medicine as a specialty. Tulane Studies in Health Policy, Working Paper #1, April 1977.

Stevens, R. The new entrepreneurialism in health care: Historical perspective. *Bull. NY Acad. Med.* 61:54–59, 1985.

Stevens, R., Goodman, L. W., and Mick, S. S. *The Alien Doctors: Foreign Medical Graduates in American Hospitals.* New York: Wiley, 1978.

Strickland, S. P. *U.S. Health Care—What's Wrong and What's Right.* New York: Universe, 1972.

Sudit, M. Self-interest or ideology? Predictors of medical students' attitudes toward health care issues. Ph.D. Dissertation, Columbia University, forthcoming.

Sumner, W. G. *Folkways.* New York: New American Library [printing used, 1960], 1906.

Sun Valley Forum on National Health. *The Foreign Medical Graduate in the U.S. Health Care System.* Monograph prepared for the Bureau of Health Manpower, DHEW, 1975.

Sussman, L. A. The personnel and ideology of public relations. *Public Opinion Q.* 12:697–708, 1948.

Szasz, T. S., and Hollander, M. H. A contribution to the philosophy of medicine: The basic models of the doctor-patient relationship. *Arch. Internal Med.* 97:585–592, 1956.

Tarlov, A. R. The increasing supply of physicians, the changing structure of the health-services system, and the future practice of medicine. *N. Engl. J. Med.* 308(20):1235–1244, 1983.

Tatalovich, R. After Medicare: Political determinants of social change in the American Medical Association. Ph.D. dissertation, University of Chicago, 1971.

Taussig, F. W., and Joslyn, C. S. *American Business Leaders: A Study in Social Origins and Social Stratification*. New York: Macmillan, 1932.

Thielens, W., Jr. Some comparisons of entrants to medical and law school. In Merton, R. K., Reader, G. G., and Kendall, P. L. (Eds.), *The Student Physician*. Cambridge: Harvard University Press, 1957, pp. 131-152.

This is the AMA. *J. Am. Med. Assoc.* 225:138-141, 1973.

Thomas, L. On the science and technology of medicine. *Daedalus* 106:35-46, 1977.

Thompson, J. D., and McEwen, W. J. Organizational goals and environment. *Am. Sociol. Rev.* 23:23-31, 1958.

Today's young doctor looks at medicine. *Medical World News* 12:34-48, April 9, 1971.

Truman, D. *The Governmental Process: Political Interests and Public Opinion*, Second Edition. New York: Knopf, 1971.

Truman, H. S. *Memoirs: Years of Trial and Hope* (Vol. II). Garden City, NY: Doubleday, 1956.

Twaddle, A. C. From medical sociology to the sociology of health. In Bottomore, T., Nowak, S., and Sokolowska, M. (Eds.), *Sociology: The State of the Art*. London: Sage Publications, 1982, pp. 323-358.

U.S. Bureau of the Census. Methodology and scores of socioeconomic status. Working Paper No. 15. Washington, DC, 1963.

U.S. Bureau of the Census. Statistical Abstract of the United States, 1982-83. 103rd Edition. Washington, DC, 1982.

U.S. Congress, House, Hearings on H.R. 4222, Health Services for the Aged, 1315, 1961.

U.S. Congress, Office of Technology Assessment. Assessing the Efficacy and Safety of Medical Technologies, OTA-H-75. Washington, D.C., Sept. 1978.

U.S. Congress, Office of Technology Assessment. Strategies for Medical Technology Assessment, OTA-H-181. Washington, D.C., Sept. 1982.

U.S. Department of Health, Education, and Welfare. Trends Affecting the U.S. Health Care System. DHEW Publ. No. HRA 76-14503. Washington, 1976.

U.S. Department of Health, Education, and Welfare. Social and Psychological Characteristics in Medical Specialty and Geographic Decisions. Hyattsville, MD: Health Resources Administration. DHEW Publ. No. HRA 78-13, 1978.

U.S. Department of Health and Human Services. *Health-United States, 1980*. Washington, D.C.: Government Printing Office, 1980.

U.S. Department of Health and Human Services. *Health-United States, 1982*. Washington, D.C.: Government Printing Office, 1982.

U.S. Department of Health and Human Services. *Health-United States, 1983*. Washington, D.C.: Government Printing Office, 1983.

U.S. Department of Health and Human Services. Private Insurance and Public Programs: Coverage of Health Services. DHHS Publication No. (PHS)85-3374, Rockville, MD, 1985.

U.S. War Department. Opinions about Negro infantry platoons in white companies of seven divisions. Report No. B-157, 1945. In Swanson, G. E., Newcomb, T. M., and Hartley, E. L. (Eds.), *Readings in Social Psychology*. Revised Edition. New York: Henry Holt, 1952. Pp. 502-506.

Unrest on the medical campus. *Medical World News* 8:63-67, Oct. 13, 1967.

Veatch, R. M. Ethical dilemmas of for-profit enterprise in health care. In Gray, B. H. (Ed.), *The New Health Care for Profit*. Washington: National Academy Press, 1983, pp. 125-152.

Vollmer, H. M., and Mills, D. L. (Eds.), *Professionalization*. Englewood Cliffs, NJ: Prentice-Hall, 1966.

Walker, N., and Argyle, M. Does the law affect moral judgments? *British J. of Criminology* 5:570–581, 1964.

Warner, W. L., and Abegglen, J. C. *Big Business Leaders in America*. New York: Harper and Brothers, 1955.

Weichert, B. C. Health care expenditures. In U.S. Department of Health and Human Services, *Health—United States, 1981*. Washington, DC: U.S. Government Printing Office, 1981.

Wentworth, W. W. *Context and Understanding: An Inquiry into Socialization Theory.* New York: Elsevier, 1980.

What doctors think of their patients. *Life*, Oct. 2, 1970, pp. 68–72.

Where doctors stand: New survey of doctors' attitudes on controversial social issues. *Hospital Physician*, Sept. 1970, pp. 49–69.

Wildavsky, A. Doing better and feeling worse: The political pathology of health policy. *Daedalus* 106:105–123, 1977.

Wilensky, H. L. The problems and prospects of the welfare state. In Wilensky, H. L. and Lebeaux, C. N. (Eds.), *Industrial Society and Social Welfare*. New York: Free Press, 1965.

Wilensky, H. L. *The Welfare State and Equality*. Berkeley: University of California Press, 1975.

Wilson, R. W., and White, E. L. Changes in morbidity, disability, and utilization differentials between the poor and non-poor: Data from the Health Interview Survey: 1964 and 1973. *Medical Care* 15(8):636–646, 1977.

Wlodkowski, B. A. Caveat emptor in health care. *Political Science Q.* 98(1):35–45, 1983.

Wohl, S. *The Medical Industrial Complex*. New York: Harmony Books, 1984.

Wolinsky, F. D. Why physicians choose different types of practice settings. *Health Services Research* 17:399–419, 1982.

Wrong, D. The oversocialized conception of man in modern sociology. *Am. Sociol. Rev.* 26:183–193, 1961.

Yankelovich, D. *The Changing Values on Campus*. New York: Washington Square Press, 1972.

Yarrow, M. R. (Ed.) Interpersonal dynamics in a desegregation process. *J. Social Issues* 14(1), 1958.

Yee, A. H., and Gage, N. L. Techniques for estimating the source and direction of influence in panel data. *Psychol. Bull.* 70:115–126, 1968.

Zuckerman, H. S. Evaluation of the literature on career choice within medicine. *Med. Care Rev.* 34:1079–1100, 1977.

Zuckerman, H. S. Industrial rationalization of a cottage industry: Multi-institutional hospital systems. *Ann. Am. Acad. of Political and Social Sciences* 468:216–230, 1983.

Index